Professional Development

A GUIDE FOR GENERAL PRACTICE

D0189072

Professional Development

A GUIDE FOR GENERAL PRACTICE

EDITED BY
Robin While
Associate Director of GP Education
Bath

Margareth Attwood
GP Project Manager
Wessex Deanery

b
Blackwell
Science

© 2000 by
Blackwell Science Ltd

Editorial Offices:
Osney Mead, Oxford OX2 OEL
25 John Street, London WC1N 2BL
23 Ainslie Place, Edinburgh EH3 6AJ
350 Main Street, Malden
    MA 02148-5018, USA
54 University Street, Carlton,
    Victoria 3053, Australia
10, rue Casimir Delavigne
    75006 Paris, France

Other Editorial Offices:
Blackwell Wissenschafts-Verlag GmbH
Kurfürstendamm 57
10707 Berlin, Germany

Blackwell Science KK
MG Kodenmacho Building
7–10 Kodenmacho Nihombashi
Chuo-ku, Tokyo 104, Japan

First published 2000

Set by Sparks Computer Solutions Ltd,
Oxford, UK
Printed and bound in the UK by MPG Books Ltd,
Bodmin, Cornwall

The Blackwell Science logo is a
trade mark of Blackwell Science Ltd,
registered at the United Kingdom
Trade Marks Registry

DISTRIBUTORS

Marston Book Services Ltd
PO Box 269
Abingdon, Oxon OX14 4YN
(*Orders*: Tel: 01235 465500
            Fax: 01235 465555)

USA
Blackwell Science, Inc
Commerce Place
350 Main Street
Malden, MA 02148-5018
(*Orders*: Tel: 800 759 6102
                 781 388 8250
        Fax: 781 388 8255)

Canada
Login Brothers Book Company
324 Saulteaux Crescent
Winnipeg, Manitoba R3J 3T2
(*Orders*: Tel: 204 837 2987)

Australia
Blackwell Science Pty Ltd
54 University Street
Carlton, Victoria 3053
(*Orders*: Tel: 3 9347 0300
        Fax: 3 9347 5001)

Catalogue records for this title
are available from the British Library
and the Library of Congress

ISBN 0-632-05629-0

For further information on
Blackwell Science, visit our website:
www.blackwell-science.com

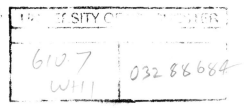

Contents

List of contributors

Dr Peter Ager
Associate GP Tutor, Westbury, Wiltshire

Mrs Margareth Attwood
Project Manager, General Practice Office, Wessex Deanery
Manager, National Office for Summative Assessment

Dr Tim Ballard RCGP
GP Trainer, Marlborough, Deputy Convenor Simulated Surgery

Dr Peter Basket
Consultant Anaesthetist, Frenchay Hospital, Bath
Editor of Resuscitation

Dr Charles Campion-Smith
GP Trainer, Dorchester

Professor Colin Coles
Educational Adviser to Wessex and South West Deaneries

Mrs Mary Connor
Senior Manager, Avon Health Authority

Mr Anthony Curtis
Senior Lecturer in Psychology, Bath Spa University College, Bath

Dr Chris Goldie
GP Trainer, Cirencester, Gloucestershire

Professor Janet Grant
Professor of Education in Medicine, Open University Institute of Educational Technology
Director of the Joint Centre for Education and Medicine

Dr Phil Hammond
GP and lecturer in Medical Communication, Bristol University Medical School
Presenter of BBC 2's Trust me I'm a Doctor

Mrs Kate Harris
Manager, Primary Care Support Unit and Practice Adviser, Wiltshire Health Authority

Professor Jacky Hayden
Dean of Postgraduate Medical Studies, North Western Deanery

Professor Roger Higgs
GP, South London
Head of Department of GP and Primary Care, King's College School of Medicine, London

Dr Claire Kendrick
GP Retainee, Bradford on Avon, Wiltshire

Dr Murray Lough
Assistant Director (Audit), West of Scotland Deanery

Mrs Lesley Millard
Head of Medical Education Development Unit at the School of Medicine, Southampton

Dr David Percy
Director of Education and Training, South East Regional Office

Dr John Pitts
Associate Director of Postgraduate GP Education – Educational Audit, Wessex Deanery

Professor Mike Pringle
Chairman RCGP, Head of Department of General Practice, Nottingham

Dr Steve Rowlands
Associate GP Tutor, Trowbridge, Wiltshire

Dr Neil Scheurmier
Primary Care Medical Adviser, Wiltshire Health Authority

Dr Frank Smith
Director of Postgraduate General Practice Education, Wessex Deanery

Dr Paul Smith
GP Trainer, Radstock, Somerset

Professor Tim van Zwanenberg
Chairman of General Practice Education Directors (COGPED)
Director of Postgraduate GP Education, Northern Deanery

Ms Sarah Walker
Clinical Quality Co-ordinator, Wiltshire Health Authority

Dr Richard Wharton
GP Tutor, Bath

Dr Robin While
Associate Director of Postgraduate GP Education, Bath
Senior Lecturer, University of Bath

Mrs Flavia Woodwark
GP Education Services Manager, Wessex Deanery

Foreword

The change from continuing medical education to continuing professional development (CPD) is challenging. It is a move away from measuring and valuing time 'bums on seats' to improved learning and better patient care.

Time spent in education is easy to measure. Yet we know that 'education' as recognized by PGEA is often not the best way to address the educational needs of general practitioners and primary-care nurses. If, for example, a doctor recognizes that he or she is not up to date in the use of drugs for the treatment of Parkinson's disease, it may be a long time before a suitable lecture comes up and even then it is unlikely to address his or her particular educational needs.

Learning is difficult to measure and cannot be demonstrated just by attending a lecture, taking part in a seminar or reading a journal. The first requirement is to identify educational need. Often this can come from reflection on one's daily clinical practice or it can follow from a discussion with a colleague. It can also come from a presentation at a conference or by attending a lecture—traditional education will live on!

Once an educational need is identified, then a responsible doctor should plan to address it. We have access to a host of reference works. We may need to look at research evidence. Colleagues may help us or we may find a course that directly meets our need. The difference is that education will be focused on meeting our need, not on some other person's perception of our need.

It is important that our learning is implemented and integrated into our clinical care. If we do this, we will improve patient care and improve ourselves as clinicians. That is the Holy Grail of CPD. It will not take more time, hopefully it will take less. But the yield per hour will be much, much greater.

A practice does not, however, operate in isolation. It must respond to national initiatives such as the National Service Frameworks, local priorities in the health improvement plan, and the needs of the practice shown through a health needs assessment. These needs should be encapsulated in a practice professional development plan (PPDP) and this plan should drive the educational process within the practice and feed into the individual practice development plans of all the members of the primary healthcare team.

That may sound complicated, but help is at hand. This excellent publication gives practical advice on how these processes can occur. It contains all the tools we need to move into continuing professional development of individuals and practice teams. It is lucid and practical; informative and developmental.

In these pages you will find a blueprint for your practice professional development plan and your personal development plan. It is a route map for CPD and life-long learning. You can't go wrong!

PROFESSOR MIKE PRINGLE
Chairman of Council, Royal College of General Practitioners

Preface

Once again the NHS is changing and along with this come changes in professional development and the introduction of revalidation. Change is stressful but offers new opportunities. This book will help to minimize the stress that you face in changing the profession's approach to improving quality in practice.

Primary healthcare teams can use this workbook as a 'hands on' practical guide to meeting the requirements of continuing professional development, clinical governance and professional revalidation. This will provide a model to replace PGEA and fit in with the development of primary-care groups and the introduction of clinical governance. It is not an exhaustive list of what can and cannot be done but a framework into which you can dovetail your own ideas.

This workbook has been largely funded by Wiltshire Health Authority and supported by the NHS Executive (Wessex Deanery). It builds on the success of the Bath Associate GP Tutor System.

Finally, we must thank all those who have helped to compile this workbook. We are grateful particularly to those who contributed chapters, responded to the draft versions and did the proof reading.

ROBIN WHILE
Associate Director of GP Education
Bath

MARGARETH ATTWOOD
GP Project Manager
Wessex Deanery

List of abbreviations

CASP	Critical Appraisal Skills Programme
CHC	Community Health Council
CHD	Coronary Heart Disease
CHIMP	Commission for Health Improvement
CMO	Chief Medical Officer
COAD	Chronic Obstructive Airways Disease
COPD	Chronic Obstructive Pulmonary Disease
CPD	Continuing Professional Development
CPR	Cardio Pulmonary Resuscitation
EBM	Evidence-Based Medicine
ECG	Electrocardiogram
ENT	Ear, Nose and Throat
GPC	General Practice Committe
HImP	Health Improvement Plan
MCQ	Multiple Choice Questionnaire
MI	Myocardial Infarction
NICE	National Institute for Clinical Excellence
NSF	National Service Framework
PACT	Prescription Analysis and Cost
PCG	Primary-Care Group
PCRN	Primary Care Research Networks
PDP	Personal Development Plan
PEP	Phased Evaluation Plan
PGEA	Postgraduate Educational Allowance
PHCT	Primary Healthcare Team
PI	Performance Indicator
PGMC	Postgraduate Medical Centre
PMS	Personal Medical Services
PPDP	Practice Professional Development Plan
R&D	Research & Development
RCGP	Royal College of General Practitioners

PART 1
Getting started

How to use this workbook

The aim of this workbook is to explain not only what the terms practice professional development plan (PPDP) and personal development plan (PDP) actually mean, but also to provide the mechanism to make them happen. General practitioners work 'at the coal-face' of delivering care to a patient population with ever increasing demands and expectations. Now, with the added demands of clinical governance and primary-care groups, it is hardly surprising that many feel overwhelmed.

This workbook aims to provide the key to meeting the requirements of a PPDP, PDP, clinical governance and revalidation all in one go. It takes a 'painting by numbers' approach, starting with health needs assessment through to the formulation of a PPDP and then, by identifying individual learning needs, to a PDP. It is a menu of opportunities, some of which may seem to be more relevant or useful than others. Each section gives some basic information together with a sample completed form and a blank form ready to be completed by the reader.

The Chief Medical Officer in *A Review of Continuing Professional Development in General Practices 1998* recommended that the key to professional development is the PPDP from which individuals could go on to develop their own PDP. Logically, this must start with a health needs assessment of the practice population, going on to look at the strengths and skill mix of the primary healthcare team (PHCT). This is a good starting point, but the PPDP should be based not only on a health needs assessment and the plans and aspirations of the practice but also on the evidence of what is going well and not so well in the practice by means of significant-event auditing, PACT data, complaints and performance indicators which will all provide the evidence to support a PPDP. There is no reason why principles underpinning evidence-based medicine should not apply to PPDPs and PDPs. It would seem sensible for a development plan to be for not less than a 5-year term.

If a PPDP is the starting point, a PDP is just as important. It is recommended that an individual PDP should relate in some way to the PPDP. If, for instance, a practice identifies a need to provide an in-house rheumatology service and no one in the PHCT has the skills and knowledge to take the lead, someone in the team would need to include it in their PDP, which could, for example, state that they were planning to study for an MSc in primary-care rheumatology by distance learning.

Each member of the PHCT should offer to become a resource for the practice by taking on something from the PPDP into his or her PDP. Non-principals (locums, assistants, retainees and GP registrars) working regularly in the practice should also be included. All team members will of course have different learning needs and plans for the future. This workbook attempts to show how these needs might be identified and discusses various methods of meeting these needs. There is also a reminder about the importance of certain generic skills, knowledge and attitudes, such as consultation skills, resuscitation, medical ethics and 'looking after your-self', which are so important for everyone who works in primary care.

A portfolio or educational log is a system by which the evidence of learning can be collected but it also provides a mechanism for external evaluation, which is likely to be important for the purposes of clinical governance and revalidation.

Finally, to quote from the *Gestalt Law of Pragnanz*, 'The whole is more than the sum of its parts'. This is surely true in primary care where the practice (the whole) is more than the sum of the individual GPs that comprise it. This should be borne in mind when formulating a PPDP. It is very important to reflect on the relationships between the parts, not just the parts themselves, in considering overall effectiveness.

The Chief Medical Officer's report

This framework for professional development was inspired by the report *A Review of Continuing Professional Development in General Practice 1998* emphasizing a high premium on quality in the NHS. The pursuit of quality can be broken down into three distinct but inter-related strands:

- clinical governance;
- enhanced professional self-regulation; and
- lifelong learning.

Clinical governance is a system through which NHS organizations are accountable for continuously improving the quality of their services and safeguarding high standards of care by creating an environment in which excellence in clinical care will flourish. Continuing professional development (CPD) is one of the central components of clinical governance and can be defined as:

> A process of lifelong learning for all individuals and teams which enables professionals to expand and fulfil their potential and which also meets the needs of patients and delivers the health and health care priorities of the NHS.

The traditional model of PGEA has fundamental weaknesses. Often the learning methods are inappropriate and the evaluation of its impact is, in general, rudimentary. There is fragmentation among different groups within primary care leading to difficulty in achieving a co-ordinated approach to education. The vision of the CMO's report identifies three interested parties: (i) the profession; (ii) the patients; and (iii) the NHS. Continuing professional development needs to be seen in this context. The concept of CPD is relatively new in the field of medicine but has been used extensively and successfully elsewhere.

What is professional development?

Right at the outset, it is important to understand what we mean by 'professional development'. Rather surprisingly, many of the interventions in recent years have not been fully thought through, nor been entirely explicit about the nature of professional practice and how it develops. Nor have they always presented the (again surprisingly large) literature that forms the evidence base for professional development. This section looks at some of the concepts involved, and presents some of the evidence. Inevitably, this discussion will be rather truncated, and if you are interested in knowing more you are advised to look at the references section (p. 176).

To try to understand professional development we will briefly try to answer four key questions:
- What is professional practice?
- What is professional knowledge?
- How does practice change naturally?
- How can natural change be fostered?

What is professional practice?

Anyone entering a profession adopts what Golby and Parrott (1999) call 'a tradition of conduct'. As Carr (1995) puts it:

> A 'practice'… is always to act within a tradition, and it is only by submitting to its authority that practitioners can begin to acquire the practical knowledge and standards of excellence by means of which their own practical competence can be judged. (pp. 68–9)

Carr claims that this form of practice:

> … can only be made intelligible in terms of the inherited and largely unarticulated body of practical knowledge which constitutes the tradition within which the good intrinsic to a practice is enshrined. (p. 68)

Epstein (1999) notes that much professional practice is 'unconscious'. Experienced clinicians, he says:

> … apply to their practice a large body of knowledge, skill, values, and experiences that are not explicitly stated by or known to them … While explicit elements of practice are taught formally, tacit elements are usually learned during observation and practice. Often excellent clinicians are less able to articulate what they do than others who observe them … Evidence-based medicine offers a structure for analysing medical decision-making, but it is not sufficient to describe the more tacit process of expert clinical judgement. (p. 834)

Professional practice means dealing with difficult, complex problems that are often 'indeterminate' (Schön 1984). It is concerned with 'the swampy lowlands' (Schön 1984), and requires 'reading the situation' (Fish & Coles 1998), being flexible, and (perhaps surprisingly for those who believe exclusively in evidence-based medicine) *improvising*.

This certainly has an implication for protocols, which are devised to determine what professionals should do in *routine* cases. What Schön is saying (and many others agree) is that the expertise of the professional comes into being *in situations where protocols can no longer apply* (which, as doctors recognize, is most of the time!).

But becoming a *caring* professional also means accepting a commitment to some form of human welfare:

> The kind of work [caring professionals] do is … especially important for the well-being of individuals or of society at large, having a value so special that money cannot serve as its sole measure; it is…Good Work. (Freidson 1994, p. 200)

What is professional knowledge?

The General Medical Council (GMC 1993) recognizes much of this when it notes that one of the attributes of the independent medical practitioner is:

> The capacity to solve clinical and other problems in medical practice, which involves or requires: (i) an intellectual and temperamental ability to change, to face the unfamiliar and to adapt to change; (ii) a capacity for individual, self-directed learning; and (iii) reasoning and judgement in the application of knowledge to the analysis and interpretation of data, in defining the nature of a problem, and in planning and implementing a strategy to resolve it. (p. 25)

Professional practice in healthcare then, is a *moral endeavour*—it fundamentally involves the capacity of someone to engage in 'right' action in human situations, where there is often no 'absolute' or 'correct' answer, only one which engages the professional in 'that form of wise and prudent judgement which takes account of what would be morally appropriate in a particular situation' (Carr 1995, pp. 70–1). Professional action can only be considered 'right' then, in the sense that it is based on 'reasoned action that can be defended discursively in argument and justified as morally appropriate to the particular circumstances in which it was taken' (Carr 1995, p. 71).

Eraut (1994) distinguishes between different kinds of professional knowledge, noting that factual (or as he calls it 'propositional') knowledge is only part of what informs professional action. Professionals also possess 'personal knowledge', which is acquired through experience.

Carr (1995) distinguishes between human actions which on the one hand lead to making something (which requires a form of knowledge the Greeks called *techne,* which today we would call 'technical knowledge'), and other forms of human action that lead to people's moral judgements, which requires a special kind of knowledge, *phronesis*, which today we would translate as 'practical wisdom'.

Professional knowledge then, is:

> … not a way of resolving technical problems for which there is, in principle, some correct answer. Rather it is a way of resolving those moral dilemmas which occur when different ethically desirable ends entail different, and perhaps incompatible, courses of action. (pp. 70–1)

How does professional practice change naturally?

Much of the practical wisdom needed for professional practice is acquired 'naturally', that is by professional people 'absorbing and being absorbed into a community of practice' (Lave & Wenger 1991). This occurs largely through the everyday conversations professionals have with one another, through them learning *from* talk as well as learning *to* talk (Lave & Wenger 1991). In short, professionals are 'socialized' into the traditions of their practice.

However, to say that professionals enter into a tradition does not imply that professional practice is merely 'passed on' uncritically from one generation to the next. It is not 'mechanically or passively reproduced' (Carr 1995, p. 69). As Carr notes 'the authoritative nature of a tradition doesn't make it immune to criticism' (p. 69). Rather, he argues, a key principle of 'being professional' is that professionals ensure that their practice is 'constantly being reinterpreted and revised through dialogue and discussion about how to pursue the practical goods which constitute the tradition' (p. 69). Epstein (1999) calls this 'mindful practice'.

Carr's argument is that this 'capacity' for changing one's practice is developed through what he calls 'critical reconstruction'. This is a process through which 'a tradition evolves and changes rather than remains static and fixed' (p. 69). He warns that someone who lacks this capacity for critical reconstruction 'may be technically accountable, but … can never be morally answerable' (p. 71). He also sees this as a corporate process where 'the collective deliberation of the many is always preferable to the isolated deliberation of the individual' (p. 71).

This implies that the caring professional is not just someone with technical expertise, nor someone capable of making prudent judgements in complex, indeterminate situations (Eraut 1994; Schön 1984) where there is a moral concern for others. It also suggests that professionals engage in the 'critical reconstruction' of their practice, that is they 'deliberate' on their practice so as to defend and justify their judgements in the light of the particular circumstances in which they were made.

This, then, clarifies the aims of professional education—it is not simply a technical updating of competence (although technical competence is important too) but a constant renewal of one's capacity to make professional judgements. Furthermore, it clarifies the fact that professional people, *because they are professionals*, seek constantly to refine their practice. Throughout their careers, doctors are learning and refining this capacity to change *through their practice.*

How can natural change be fostered?

So, change is natural for professionals, but it does not always happen. Why is this? A Standing Committee on Postgraduate Medical and Dental Education (SCOPME) report (1998a) on continuing professional development suggested a number of reasons:

- pressures of service work;
- inappropriate work tasks;
- education not being valued or rewarded;
- no feedback or review (SCOPME 1999); and
- the Colleges' points systems.

Clearly, then, any new CPD interventions must not merely reinvent the same wonky wheel! But what *should* happen? SCOPME suggests the following:

- people's needs must be voiced;
- a balance of personal, professional and work;
- development should be recognized and valued;
- there should be the local analysis of problems and solutions;
- mentor's skills need developing (SCOPME 1998b);
- CPD schemes should be evaluated;
- CPD should not be related to monitoring, accreditation, remuneration or promotion; and
- organizational support should be given.

Further insight comes from the Government's White Paper on quality *A First Class Service* (NHS 1998). In its definition of 'clinical governance' there is the following suggestion as to how quality can be established:

... by creating an environment in which excellence in health care will flourish. (NHS 1998, p. 33)

There is in this phrase a biological, even botanical, imagery. We all know about environments that lead to things flourishing: there is nurturing, nutrients, warmth, support. (We also know about environments where things do not flourish: these are deserts, hostile, overcrowded, lacking in basic life support.)

Natural development is more likely to occur in a supportive environment, and CPD arrangements should facilitate this. This workbook seeks to meet this objective.

Where do we start?

The practice professional development plan (PPDP)

In the past, GP and practice education has tended to be haphazard, often shaped by other people's perceptions of our needs. This method is refreshingly different, putting you and your practice at the centre of the learning process. The aim of this workbook is to enable you to identify your learning and development priorities. It also deals with how to collect the evidence of learning and discusses the 'Use of portfolios in learning'.

For education and learning to be effective it needs to be appropriate, both for our patients and ourselves. At the heart of the PPDP is the assessment of both of these elements. No two practices are the same and every practice plan will be subtly, or dramatically, different from another's. It may be appropriate to build into this plan the needs of the primary-care group (PCG).

To start with, a practice will need to assess the health needs of its patients (this sounds more daunting than it really is). It will need to involve the whole team in looking at individuals' strengths, weaknesses and learning styles. Subsequently, it can identify its development priorities, which can be considered alongside the health needs of its patients.

This workbook provides a step-by-step guide to achieving and recording a development plan uniquely tailored to your needs and the needs of your practice. It will help you to work out your aims and objectives over the following years, as well as how and when you plan to achieve them.

This development plan needs to be owned jointly by the members of the practice and not imposed by one individual. To ensure success, members of the team will need to feel that they have contributed to the PPDP and that it belongs to them.

The personal development plan (PDP)

When you take the decision to develop your own personal development plan (PDP), begin by writing down your aims and objectives.
- What do you want to achieve over the next 5 years?
- Which specific things need to be done to achieve it?
- How and when are these specific things going to be tackled?

This workbook illustrates a number of methods by which learning needs can be identified. An important theme that emerges is the development of reflective practice.

The PPDP gives you the strategic direction for education and development. Personal development plans are formed by combining the needs of the practice with the needs, interest and aspirations of you as an individual. This book provides an opportunity for professional development to become an exciting and dynamic process, which is learner centred, based on wants and needs and gives an opportunity to develop a culture of life-long learning.

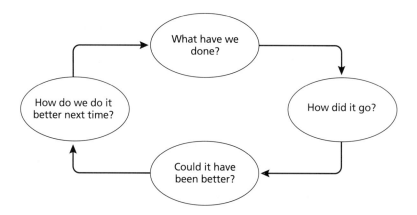

What are the best ways to learn?

There are many different styles of learning, some more enjoyable than others. There is no one method or technique that is best. GPs are unique professionals and you may have developed your own preferred style of learning, which may include reading, reflecting, planning and doing. As GPs we tend to learn best when we reflect on our practice (a pro forma to help you with this can be found on p. 12). Reflective practice is often at its most powerful when examining significant events (see p. 60). If you are unsure about your own personal learning style, further information is given on page 44.

Even when educational needs are met, such positive experiences may not feed back into practice because of various barriers (e.g. time, cost or opportunity). The challenge here is to make CPD work by ensuring that educational events produce demonstrable clinical effects. Adopting an ongoing system of monitoring and appraisal will also ensure that progress and development can be measured, further enhancing professional development.

We should remember that GP education can be intrinsically rewarding and fun!

There is a clear need to develop an ongoing practical system of managed education for primary care that is based on a needs assessment, is practice linked, and responds to both the needs of doctors and the NHS.

This workbook is designed to do exactly this: it is flexible, allows you to use your own preferred learning style, and it will enable you to assess the impact of your education on the care of your patients.

The use of portfolios in learning

A portfolio of learning is a collection of evidence that learning has taken place. It is a physical product of the learning process and gives documentary proof of learning.

To build a portfolio you need to:

1   Identify what you are seeking to learn. (This may change over time and that is fine; changes will need to be documented.)
2   Decide how you can achieve your goals, e.g. by reading, attending lectures, visiting a particular organization or using a new computer program.
3   Document the learning you achieve.
4   Write reflectively and critically about your learning experiences and their outcomes (an audiotape would be an alternative to writing but it must still be both reflective and critical).

A personal diary or log may be part of your portfolio. Indeed, this is often an exceedingly valuable way of recording and commenting on your thoughts and feelings. If you wish to use your portfolio, for example, for accreditation or to offer an interview panel, you may wish to remove these more personal documents. If your portfolio is not going to be seen by anyone else you can, of course, include whatever you choose. In both cases, the notes are merely a guide to what may be involved in building a portfolio.

In order to achieve steps 3 and 4 you might, for example, put the following into your portfolio:

- notes of a lecture you attended on the topic you wish to learn about;
- a tape recording and commentary on a radio programme on teaching or on a medical topic;
- a list of new ideas you have gained from the above activities to use in your teaching or gained in your work with patients; and
- an analysis of how well the ideas worked, what helped and hindered the changes you made, how the students or patients reacted to your new approach.

The analysis is a key part of the documentation of your learning (see figure).

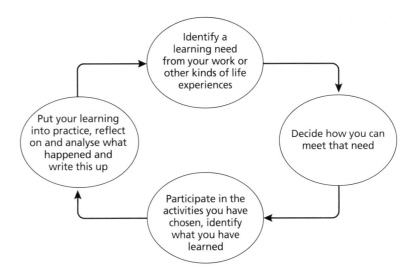

REFLECTIVE PRACTICE

Event: Communications skills workshop	Date: September 1999

What were my personal learning objectives for this event?

Benchmark my consultation skills

Learning to keep to time in surgery

Were they met?

Yes! exceeded my expectations

What important learning points have I taken away from today?

Most doctors find many consultations challenging

Being 'patient centred' need not be slower

Reflecting and summarizing

Effective ways to end consultation

What changes, if any, will I make to my practice as a result of my learning?

All booked appointments for 10 minutes

Have a free appointment every hour to allow to catch up or have a break

What is my action plan to achieve these changes?

Agenda item next practice meeting

Discuss at away day

Buy video and record some of my surgeries

My areas for improvement are:

Listening, reflecting, challenging and summarizing

My action plan for this is:

Video and view a morning surgery

Ring postgraduate tutor to find someone to help

The forces I see helping me are:

One of my partners is a trainer and able to help with videoing

To achieve this plan I need to negotiate with, and have help from:

Reception staff, manager and colleagues

To achieve this plan I need to change:

Appointment time

Introduce protocol for videoing consultations and patients' consent

I will assess my success by:

Audit of running late and review of video consultations

REVIEW

Date: 6th January 2000

What changes did I make as a result of using the action plan?

Better time keeping and now more effective at ending consultations

What have I learnt from this?

That I am able to change and that I am in control!

HOW HAS IT BENEFITED:

My patients	My staff	Myself
Are less irritated about being kept waiting	Are getting less flak from patients	I am less stressed

When will I further review progress?

6/12 to check consultation style and time keeping

REFLECTIVE PRACTICE

Event:	Date:

What were my personal learning objectives for this event?

Were they met?

What important learning points have I taken away from today?

What changes, if any, will I make to my practice as a result of my learning?

What is my action plan to achieve these changes?

My areas for improvement are:

My action plan for this is:

The forces I see helping me are:

To achieve this plan I need to negotiate with, and have help from:

To achieve this plan I need to change:

I will assess my success by:

REVIEW

Date:

What changes did I make as a result of using the action plan?

What have I learnt from this?

HOW HAS IT BENEFITED:

My patients	My staff	Myself

When will I further review progress?

PART 2

Practice Professional Development

Health needs assessment

What is health needs assessment?
It is a judgement formed by the understanding of a population's benefit in terms of health gain, ranging from provision of services through to prevention and palliative care.

It is an understanding of a population's benefit in terms of health gain based on a knowledge of:
- incidence and prevalence of diseases;
- effective intervention; and
- a profile of the population studied.

What are its benefits?
It enables you to identify the needs of your practice population and set and prioritize both the short- and long-term objectives which will be the basis of your practice professional development plan (PPDP).

It also:
- provides a method of sifting through endless priorities;
- focuses attention on key tasks;
- gives a degree of control and ownership through choosing priorities and targets;
- allows the creation of an action plan to achieve these objectives which will then form the basis for your PPDP; and
- puts teamworking skills into practice.

What is involved?
1 Creating a profile of your practice population (see p. 20).
2 Identification of key features of your practice population (see p. 22).
3 Identification of top health problems in your practice (see p. 24).
4 Prioritizing the list (see p. 28).
5 Planning interventions (see p. 30).
6 Creating an action plan (see p. 34).
7 New priorities (see p. 36).

Your local health authority may be able to help you with necessary statistics.

1 CREATING A PROFILE OF YOUR PRACTICE POPULATION

PRACTICE AREA

Urban/rural or mixed	Mixed
Demographic features	11% of practice population have chronic illness High proportion of one-parent families
Employment/unemployment levels	Low unemployment
Local employers	Westinghouse, light industry, agricultural, commuters to Bath, Bristol and London
Access to services (i.e. transport facilities)	One in five has no car, poor public transport Village link operates
What is it like to live here?	Some rural poverty but mostly middle class and affluent, nice countryside but can be isolated. Very good doctors!

The age/sex spread of the practice population

Age groups	0–4	5–16	17–24	25–34	35–44	45–54	55–64	65–74	75–84	85–89	90+
Males	101	266	135	245	338	314	206	181	71	13	6
Females	130	288	118	296	315	308	202	161	110	26	17
Total both sexes	231	554	253	541	653	622	408	342	181	39	23

Figures from age/sex register on (date)

05/08/99

Population trends:

March 1995	3487
March 1996	3553
March 1997	3612
March 1998	3759
March 1999	3850

Is your population increasing or decreasing?

Increasing slowly

What are the reasons?

New housing development

1 CREATING A PROFILE OF YOUR PRACTICE POPULATION

PRACTICE AREA

Urban/rural or mixed	
Demographic features	
Employment/unemployment levels	
Local employers	
Access to services (i.e. transport facilities)	
What is it like to live here?	

The age/sex spread of the practice population

Age groups	0–4	5–16	17–24	25–34	35–44	45–54	55–64	65–74	75–84	85–89	90+
Males											
Females											
Total both sexes											

Figures from age/sex register on (date)

Population trends:

March 1995	
March 1996	
March 1997	
March 1998	
March 1999	

Is your population increasing or decreasing?

What are the reasons?

2 KEY FEATURES OF YOUR PRACTICE POPULATION

When looking at your practice population always view it with an eye to pick up features you are able to influence. Be specific rather than general, very broad areas are difficult to tackle.

Causes of substantial mortality

Coronary heart disease

Cancer

Stroke

Causes of substantial ill-health

Smoking

Asthma

Ischaemic heart disease

Hypertension

Obesity

Diabetes

Areas of concern

High rates of hospitalization

Substance dependency

Health needs of 15–24 year olds

Accidents: under 5s

Accidents: over 75s

Dignity and comfort for the terminally ill

Support for carers

Other considerations

HImP

Priorities of PCG

When looking at your practice population always view it with an eye to pick up features you are able to influence. Be specific rather than general, very broad areas are difficult to tackle.

2 KEY FEATURES OF YOUR PRACTICE POPULATION

Causes of substantial mortality

Causes of substantial ill-health

Areas of concern

Other considerations

3 IDENTIFICATION OF TOP HEALTH PROBLEMS IN YOUR PRACTICE

List the top health problems in your practice. These may include priorities that you can influence directly, or priorities on which you might have to work with others, e.g. voluntary organizations, social services, local schools, etc.

Involve the whole team in completing the questionnaire on the following pages.

Take into account:
- national priorities, e.g. 'Our Healthier Nation';
- health authority priorities, e.g. Director of Public Health's annual report;
- primary-care groups;
- local priorities:
  practice disease and morbidity register
  primary-care team's knowledge
  philosophy of the practice.

---

1 Description of the practice population

High elderly population

Rural occupations—farming community

Low unemployment

Predominantly middle class

Limited public transport/poor access to services

Commuters

---

2 Based on our own experience, are there key things that stick out as health problems in our practice?

Elderly isolated

Commuters—work in London, live in Wiltshire

    (unable to attend surgery appointments)

Diabetes

Asthma admissions

Coronary heart disease

Prevalence of depression seems low

    Are we missing something?

Dependence on health services

---

3 How do you think these differ from other areas/practices?

Predominantly middle class—healthcare dependency

Rural/isolated areas

High elderly population

4 What things help people feel healthy here?

Fresh air/pleasant, friendly environment/
rural, picturesque countryside

Caring services

Good housing

Supportive neighbours

Access to sport centres and gyms

Exercise

5 What stops people feeling healthy?

Isolation

Access to surgery

Access to services (e.g. social services, NHS)

Access to shops

Motorways

Pylons!

6 Are there key things that could be done to improve people's health?

Improve public transport

Advise about accident prevention and
healthy lifestyles

Access to link worker

More effective use of health visitor

Access to surgery

7 Are there key things the practice could do to improve people's health?

Improve care of chronic disease, diabetes, COAD

Opportunistic advice about life styles

Opportunistic screening re family histories

Extend surgery hours to provide appointments
for commuters

More nurse-led chronic disease management clinics

Smoke stop clinics

25

3 IDENTIFICATION OF TOP HEALTH PROBLEMS IN YOUR PRACTICE

1 Description of the practice population

2 Based on our own experience, are there key things that stick out as health problems in our practice?

3 How do you think these differ from other areas/practices?

4 What things help people feel healthy here?

5 What stops people feeling healthy?

6 Are there key things that could be done to improve people's health?

7 Are there key things the practice could do to improve people's health?

4 PRIORITIZING THE LIST

Involve the primary-care team in choosing criteria to prioritize the list, e.g. effectiveness of interventions, recognizable benefits to the community.

Apply your chosen criteria to select three or four areas on which to focus attention in the following year.

Ask the following questions of each health need identified	HEALTH NEEDS		
	Can we improve our prevention of coronary heart disease?	Can we improve the care of patients with asthma?	Can we improve our care for housebound diabetic patients?
1 Interest to whole team	4	3	4
2 Achievable with available resources	4	4	4
3 Easily identified group	4	4	4
4 Recognizable benefits to the community team	4	4	4
5 Effectiveness of interventions, e.g. health outcomes	4	4	2
6 Worth doing something about—prevalence	4	4	4
7 How much energy is needed	4	4	4
8 Importance to community	4	4	4
Total			

As a result of this exercise what are we going to choose to go onto our PPDP?
Secondary prevention of coronary heart disease

0 = Does not meet criteria 1 2 3 4 = Meets criteria

4 PRIORITIZING THE LIST

Involve the primary-care team in choosing criteria to prioritize the list, e.g. effectiveness of interventions, recognizable benefits to the community.

Apply your chosen criteria to select three or four areas on which to focus attention in the following year.

Ask the following questions of each health need identified	HEALTH NEEDS		
	Can we improve our prevention of coronary heart disease?	Can we improve the care of patients with asthma?	Can we improve our care for housebound diabetic patients?
1 Interest to whole team			
2 Achievable with available resources			
3 Easily identified group			
4 Recognizable benefits to the community team			
5 Effectiveness of interventions, e.g. health outcomes			
6 Worth doing something about—prevalence			
7 How much energy is needed			
8 Importance to community			
Total			

As a result of this exercise what are we going to choose to go onto our PPDP?

0 = Does not meet criteria
1
2
3
4 = Meets criteria

5 PLANNING INTERVENTIONS

HEALTH PROBLEM

Secondary prevention of coronary heart disease

CHECKING OUT ASSUMPTIONS

What information do we have on this health problem?

Fairly complete but need to review similar read-coded diagnoses, e.g. angina, MI, history of MI, ischaemic heart disease, etc.

Majority of computer templates complete

How accessible is the information, e.g. paper notes, on computer?

Information on computer EMIS Version 4. Fairly accessible but not always accurate.

What information might we need to collect in the future?

Need to ensure that computer templates are complete and agree

1 read-codes for coronary heart disease

2 protocol for accuracy of data entry

Information should include weight, BMI, smoking, diabetes, family history, blood pressure, cholesterol and exercise

COLLECTING INFORMATION

How easy is it to extract information, e.g. prescribing referrals, risk factors?

1 Run computer search on read-codes or key word, e.g. angina

2 Try running search on prescribing information, e.g. statin or aspirin

Do we wish to set up systems to collect other necessary information?

1 ? Pilot use of MIQUEST

2 Ensure accuracy of data by medical staff (this is key!)

'You are only as good as your weakest link'

What services are currently provided for this health problem?

Clinics, with data entered on evidence-based computer templates

If services are currently provided who provides them?

Doctors and nurses

What are appropriate interventions for this problem?

Cholesterol measurement

Advice re life style, and treatment with aspirin, anticoagulation and statins

What might we provide in the practice differently to meet this health need?

Develop recall system for non-attenders

What other resources can we tap into?

More use of health visitor

Sports centre for graded exercise prescription

How will we know that things have improved?

Clinical audit against key markers, e.g. cholesterol, aspirin and statins, etc.

5 PLANNING INTERVENTIONS

HEALTH PROBLEM

CHECKING OUT ASSUMPTIONS

> **What information do we have on this health problem?**

> **How accessible is the information, e.g. paper notes, on computer?**

> **What information might we need to collect in the future?**

COLLECTING INFORMATION

> **How easy is it to extract information, e.g. prescribing referrals, risk factors?**

> **Do we wish to set up systems to collect other necessary information?**

> **What services are currently provided for this health problem?**

If services are currently provided who provides them?

What are appropriate interventions for this problem?

What might we provide in the practice differently to meet this health need?

What other resources can we tap into?

How will we know that things have improved?

6 CREATING AN ACTION PLAN

Who will be involved?

Clinical staff supported by administrative staff

How will they do it?

Ensure accuracy of disease register currently held on EMIS Version 4

Baseline assessment to see where we are now

Establish evidence-based computer template for secondary prevention chronic heart disease

Generate recall letters, advising patients that the practice would like to review them every 6 months

Record attendance with results of investigations and examination findings on computer template

Audit of non-attenders every 3 months with reminder letters sent

Annual audit of clinical effectiveness against key markers, e.g. diastolic blood pressure, smoking, cholesterol, BMI, exercise, aspirin, etc.

By when?

Priority year 1

EVALUATION

What was successful?

Disease register for coronary heart disease sorted out

98% of target group had blood pressure checked and smoking status recorded

Cholesterol fallen over year and all patients without contra-indications were on aspirin

What was not so successful and why?

Percentage of smokers still the same (smoke stop clinic on Monday morning)

What might we do differently in future?

Rationalize our statin prescribing

Arrange a more convenient smoke stop clinic

6 CREATING AN ACTION PLAN

Who will be involved?

How will they do it?

By when?

EVALUATION

What was successful?

What was not so successful and why?

What might we do differently in future?

7 NEW PRIORITIES

> *Once we have 'cracked' coronary heart disease, we plan to do the same for asthma, COAD and diabetes mellitus.*

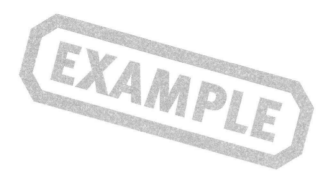

You can continually build on your practice's original health needs assessment by evaluating whether you should continue with the same priorities on a longer-term basis, or set new priorities for the following year. This should be completed in conjunction with your PPDP and be part of your annual planning cycle.

7 NEW PRIORITIES

You can continually build on your practice's original health needs assessment by evaluating whether you should continue with the same priorities on a longer-term basis, or set new priorities for the following year. This should be completed in conjunction with your PPDP and be part of your annual planning cycle.

The primary healthcare team

The away day/protected time approach to professional development
What are away days?

Away days or half-day get-togethers for entire practices, although still a relatively new idea, are on the increase. With some forward planning (being certain to tell your patients well beforehand, and leaving notices giving them the alternative instructions), you can arrange for a nearby practice to cover for the day or half-day. You, your staff and attached community staff can then have some relaxed reflective time determining future strategy for your practice. Do not forget to include any regular non-principals attached to the practice in the away day process. If they and other staff are unable to attend, a feedback session after the event would be helpful.

Why have them?

Away days can be used to bring together various pieces of work in order to agree as a team on the priorities for the coming year.

What can be achieved?

- Identification of clinical and organizational priorities.
- Identification of skills to meet these priorities.
- Identification of gaps and overlaps in service provision.
- Recommendations for addressing the gaps and overlaps in provision.

An example of a practice away day programme is shown on the opposite page, followed by ground rules and helpful information on running small groups.

AWAY DAY PROGRAMME

9.30 a.m.
Part One: Welcome and expectations
Theme:
Where are we now?
Where do we want to be?
How are we going to get there?

Ground rules
Ice breaker: Learning styles (see p. 44)

10.30 a.m.
Part Two: Where are we now?
Practice SCOT (strengths, challenges, opportunities, threats)
   analysis (see p. 43)
What has gone well?
What could we do better?
What could we improve upon?

12.15 p.m. Lunch

'Vision for the Future'

1.00 p.m.
Part Three: Where do we want to be?
Pairs/group brainstorm (see p. 41)
What gets in the way?
What are the solutions?

3.00 p.m.
Part Four: How are we going to get there?
• Discuss, agree and prioritize the PPDP
• Identification of key action areas for individuals or team
• Action plan—who does what? by when?
• Date of review

4.30 p.m.
Reflection on the day and close

Ground rules for away days

- Listen to each other, do not interrupt, give opportunities for all to contribute, show you are listening and respect the other members of the group.
- Confidentiality.
- Personal honesty.
- Be honest in a constructive way.
- Be open.
- Keep to the point.
- Keep it simple/no jargon.
- Make your own statements.
- Do not be too ambitious.
- Finish on time.

What do you want from today?

The following pointers might be helpful:

- clarity about the way forward as a PHCT;
- strengthen the PHCT;
- provide a shared understanding of the PHCT;
- establish where we are starting from;
- feel more part of the team;
- feel that as a team we are aiming at same goals (know what the goals are);
- share the barriers;
- form a vision/practice plan;
- allow the opportunity to develop a shared vision—practice development and individual needs—produce something tangible;
- time to develop personally; and
- individual development needs/skills.

Running small groups

In this type of activity the group relies principally on its own members as resources and will meet several times to cover a topic in various sections. Take, for example, *palliative care* or *chronic disease management*. There would be an aim, say, '*to improve the care of patients with chronic disease.*' This would best be broken down into objectives.

- To increase the number of post-myocardial infarction (post-MI) patients taking aspirin.
- To increase the number of post-MI patients taking a statin.
- To ensure all patients with chronic obstructive airway disease (COAD) have a maximal peak expiratory flow (PEF) recorded.
- To ensure all patients with diabetes have annual retinal screening.

Remember that an aim is a vague expression of intent, and an objective is measurable and subsequently open to audit.

'SMART' can be a useful mnemonic:
Specific, Measurable, Agreed, Reliable, And Timely.

Small groups can be exceptionally inventive, effective, cohesive and collaborative. Equally, they can be uncomfortable, acrimonious and emotionally fraught. Good leadership will enhance the possibilities for success and reduce the risk of disaster. Most people, but not all, can work in small groups.

Tips on running small groups

• The group should have constant membership of between five and 13, the ideal being about eight.
• Ensure all group members know each other or introduce themselves.
• All members to have equal rank (no doctors and nurses, just people with special skills, knowledge or attitude).
• The task should be agreed and clarified.
• Do not have two conversations at one time.
• Allow everyone to speak without interruption.
• Encourage the noisy to 'tone down'.
• Encourage the quiet to 'switch on'; they are used to being ignored, let them feel their opinion is as important as anyone's.
• Encourage honesty.
• Gently discourage boastfulness.
• No 'telling tales out of school'; whatever is said in a group must be confidential.
• Provide emotional support when appropriate.
• Give intellectual challenges when appropriate.
• Value openly each member's contribution.

Brainstorming

Purpose

• To increase creative skills.
• To provide a useful technique for team problem solving.

This activity helps to clarify personal goals, improve problem-solving skills, increase creativity and develop team-building skills.

Method

The technique of brainstorming can be applied in many ways. The activity can be modified to suit different needs because it is the basic method that is important. To obtain the best results, it is important to follow the rules as closely as possible.

1 Set aside at least half an hour for the activity.

2 Decide on a subject in which change and/or creativity are important. This should be a topic of interest or importance to the group. The topic should be stated as a problem, question or objective.

3 Explain that 'brainstorming' is a process in which all members of the group are invited to suggest as many ideas as they can. Make it clear that *all* ideas, no matter how absurd they may appear, will be recorded and that there will be no evaluation of the ideas during the first stage; as soon as an idea is introduced, it will be recorded, and the next idea will be introduced.

4 When everyone understands the guidelines, allow some time for the participants to ask questions. Then begin the brainstorming session by writing the chosen topic clearly on the flip chart, e.g. How can we improve communication between members of the PHCT?

5 Have the members brainstorm the topic for at least 5 minutes and list (without any discussion) *every* idea suggested. Two or three flip charts may be used to record ideas, which are likely to come thick and fast when there is a rule prohibiting evaluation or censorship.

6 Divide the participants into two groups and ask each group to decide which suggestion falls into each of two categories: 'Very Relevant' and 'Potentially Relevant'. Allow up to half an hour for this task.

7 Ask each group to list all the '*Very Relevant*' ideas on one sheet and all the '*Potentially Relevant*' ideas on a second sheet.

8 Have the groups meet together and share their lists. Ask individuals to examine the lists and to choose the suggestions that could make the greatest contribution to solving the problem or achieving the objective.

9 Take the suggestions with the highest scores and produce a written plan to implement them. (The example on the next page may help.)

10 After a suitable period of time, during which implementation is tried, have the group meet again to discuss how well the plans are progressing and to take any necessary corrective action.

BRAINSTORMING

Topic	Action steps
How can we improve communication between members of the PHCT?	PHCT meeting every month in protected time. 1 Alternate Wednesday and Friday afternoons employ locum to cover GMS 2 Each and every patient contact to be recorded on computer • surgery appointments • home visits • telephone calls • any discussion between members of PHCT 3 Copy internal e-mail to keep everyone informed

Practice SCOT analysis

Strengths and challenges are things that exist for you and your practice at this moment. Opportunities and threats are possibilities which may come along in the future, but which need to be thought about now.

You will need to maximize your strengths and opportunities and minimize your challenges and threats.

Developing a SCOT analysis could involve individual or all members of the practice team.

- **Strengths** relate to achievements over the year.
- **Challenges** highlight any difficulties or obstacles which have been experienced.
- **Opportunities** lists factors which will influence the success of individuals, team and practice, i.e. ideas for the future.
- **Threats** lists things which may be an obstacle to development.

An example could be:

Strengths	Challenges
1 Stable patient population 2 Hard working and effective PHCT 3 Dispensing 4 Paperless practice	1 Demanding patients 2 Elderly list 3 Appointments with multiple problems 4 Prevalence of chronic disease 5 Rural isolation

Opportunities	Threats
1 PMS pilots 2 Dispensing formulary 3 Integrated nursing team 4 Partners work ouside GMS, e.g. sports medicine, police, clinical assistant	1 Not enough appointment time 2 Increase in list size 3 Workload 4 Burnout

Learning profiles for primary healthcare teams
Developing a learning profile

This will:
- enable the team to learn together for the benefit of patients and themselves;
- develop consistent standards for patient care;
- build professional confidence; and
- enable team members to articulate their achievements.

What can you do for your team?

- Actively seek opportunities to learn together, i.e. have regular clinical meetings, encourage *Significant-event auditing* (see p. 60) and promote multi-disciplinary review of clinical practice.
- Encourage everyone to discover their own learning style. Information on how to obtain Honey and Mumford's *Manual of Learning Styles* and Learning Styles Questionnaire can be found below.
- Encourage everyone to reflect on their particular learning style. Try completing the *Reflecting on Learning Styles* pro forma on page 46.

The Manual of Learning Styles

Given the same experience, why do some people learn while others do not? A major reason is that people differ in the way they prefer to learn.

The Manual of Learning Styles (Honey & Mumford 1986) includes:
- Description of the learning cycle and the four styles: activist, reflector, theorist and pragmatist, for further information on the four styles see below.
- The Learning Styles Questionnaire which enables people to identify their preferred style(s).
- A variety of norms against which results can be compared.
- Suggestions on how trainers can use the information to:
  design events to cover the complete learning cycle;
  select activities to suit different preferences; and
  help individuals to strengthen under-utilized styles.
- Suggestions on how people can better manage their learning.

Each manual costs £60.00 and comes complete with a master copy of the questionnaire and score key, both of which can be photocopied.

For further information on *The Manual of Learning Styles*, Personal Workbooks and Learning Logs, contact Peter Honey Publications, Ardingly House, 10 Linden Avenue, Maidenhead, Berks, SL6 6HB (Tel 01628 633946; Fax 01628 633262; e-mail peterhoney@peterhoney.co.uk).

Learning styles: general descriptions
Activists

Activists involve themselves fully and without bias in new experiences. They enjoy the 'here and now' and are happy to be dominated by immediate experiences. They are open-minded and not sceptical, which tends to make them enthusiastic about anything new. Their philosophy is: 'I'll try anything once'. They tend to act first and consider the consequences afterwards. Their days are filled with activity. They tackle problems by brainstorming. As soon as the excitement from one activity has died down they are busy looking for the next. They tend to thrive on the challenge of new experiences but are bored with implementation and longer-term consolidation. They are gregarious people constantly involving themselves with others, but in doing so they seek to centre all activities on themselves.

Reflectors

Reflectors like to stand back to ponder experiences and observe from many different perspectives. They collect data, both first-hand and from others, and prefer to think about it thoroughly before coming to any conclusion. The thorough collection and analysis of data about experiences and events are what counts so they tend to postpone reaching definitive conclusions for as long as possible. Their philosophy is to be cautious. They are thoughtful people who like to consider all possible angles and implications before making a move. They prefer to take a back seat in meetings and discussions. They enjoy observing other people in action. They listen to others and get the drift of the discussion before making their own points. They tend to adopt a low profile and have a slightly distant, tolerant, unruffled air about them. When they act it is part of a wide picture which includes the past as well as the present and others' observations as well as their own.

Theorists

Theorists adapt and integrate observations into complex but logically sound theories. They think problems through in a vertical, step-by-step logical way. They assimilate disparate facts into coherent theories. They tend to be perfectionists who will not rest easy until things are tidy and fit into a rational scheme. They like to analyse and synthesize. They are keen on basic assumptions, principles, theories, models and systems thinking. Their philosophy prizes rationality and logic. 'If it's logical it's good.' Questions they frequently ask are: 'Does it make sense?' 'How does this fit with that?' 'What are the basic assumptions?' They tend to be detached, analytical and dedicated to rational objectivity rather than anything subjective or ambiguous. Their approach to problems is consistently logical. This is their 'mental set' and they rigidly reject anything that does not fit within it. They prefer to maximize certainty and feel uncomfortable with subjective judgements, lateral thinking and anything flippant.

Pragmatists

Pragmatists are keen on trying out ideas, theories and techniques to see if they work in practice. They positively search out new ideas and take the first opportunity to experiment with applications. They are the sort of people who return from management courses brimming with new ideas that they want to try out in practice. They like to get on with things and act quickly and confidently on ideas that attract them. They tend to be impatient with ruminating and open-ended discussions. They are essentially practical, down-to-earth people who like making practical decisions and solving problems. They respond to problems and opportunities 'as a challenge'. Their philosophy is 'There is always a better way' and 'If it works it's good'.

REFLECTING ON LEARNING STYLES QUESTIONNAIRE

Now reflect on your particular learning style (are you an activist, reflector, theorist or pragmatist?).

Give an example of how your learning style may influence an aspect of decision making in your practice

Using knowledge of this learning style what may be the best way to present an educational event that would maximize your learning and enjoyment?

Do you consider this to be true of your practice in general?

What does this preferred learning style suggest about the way you respond to changes in general practice?

Can you give a recent example of this?

How do you describe the preferred learning style of your practice?

Does this differ from your individual learning style?

If so, how might a compromise be reached in terms of an effective provision of an educational event for your practice?

Skill mix of the primary healthcare team

Skill mix is 'identifying the range of tasks and responsibilities involved in providing care within a particular speciality, what levels are involved and therefore who is appropriate to carry them out'.

The skill mix review of your current team can help once you have identified your priorities. Ask each person to measure their skills on the standards for assessment competence scale 'novice to expert' (Benner 1984).

Level 1	Novice—no knowledge or working experience.
Level 2	Advanced beginner—some knowledge and limited working experience. Needs help in setting priorities. Can demonstrate marginally acceptable performance.
Level 3	Competent—conscious deliberate planning is characteristic of this skill level. Becoming skilled but lacks the speed and flexibility to be totally proficient.
Level 4	Proficient—has an experience-based ability to recognize whole situations and therefore knows when the expected normal does not occur and modifies responses accordingly.
Level 5	Expert—enormous background knowledge and significant level of skill. Homes in on the nature of the problem without wasting time on unfruitful alternative diagnoses and solutions. May use analytic tools when the need to generate alternative perspectives (creativity) is needed.

INDIVIDUAL SKILLS ASSESSMENT

Name:

Dr P Spoons

Post:

GP Partner

Core skills	Level 1	Level 2	Level 3	Level 4	Level 5
Consultation skills					✓
Diagnosis					✓
Treatment					✓
Special interests					
Paediatrics				✓	
Cardiology			✓		
Gastroenterology				✓	
Specialist skills					
Child health surveillance					✓
Echocardiograms				✓	
Gastroscopy					✓
Flexible sigmoidoscopy				✓	

INDIVIDUAL SKILLS ASSESSMENT

Name:

Post:

Core skills	Level 1	Level 2	Level 3	Level 4	Level 5
Special interests					
Specialist skills					

TEAM SKILLS ASSESSMENT

Name of team member	Core skills and special interests	Specialist skills	Level of specialist skills				
			1	2	3	4	5
GP 1	Generic general practice	Asthma					✓
	Paediatrics	Child health surveillance					✓
	General medicine	Diabetes			✓		
		Cardiology				✓	
		Epilepsy			✓		
GP 2	Generic general practice						✓
	Obstetrics and gynaecology	Ultrasound				✓	
		Pipelle sampling				✓	
		Colposcopy				✓	
	Gastroenterology	Sigmoidoscopy					✓
GP 3	Generic general practice						✓
	Surgery	Minor surgery				✓	
	Psychiatry	Section 12 approved				✓	
		Counselling				✓	

Name of team member	Core skills and special interests	Specialist skills	Level of specialist skills				
			1	2	3	4	5
Practice nurse	Generic nursing skills	Travel vaccinations					✓
		Family planning				✓	
	Chronic disease management	Diabetes				✓	
		Hypertension				✓	
		Asthma			✓		
Community nurse	Generic community nursing skills	Wound management					✓
		Treatment of leg ulcers				✓	
		Infection control				✓	
	ITU bank nurse	High-dependency patients			✓		
Community nurse	General community nursing skills						✓
	Macmillan trained	Palliative care					✓
	ex-Urology ward sister	Continence advice				✓	
Health visitor	Generic nursing and health visitor skills	Child development				✓	
		Accident prevention			✓		
		Health education					✓
	MSc in Education	Teaching					✓
		Nurse mentor				✓	

TEAM SKILLS ASSESSMENT

Name of team member	Core skills and special interests	Specialist skills	Level of specialist skills				
			1	2	3	4	5

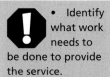

- Identify what work needs to be done to provide the service.
- Define the work that needs to be done to provide the service.
- Determine what responsibilities must be adopted and what tasks done to perform this work well and economically and to achieve specific outcomes.
- Define what mix of general skills and specific skills are required to perform to that level.

- Do the skills required fit with the needs of your patients?
- Are there any skills gaps?
- Who in the team has the potential to fill them?
- Would you like to add this to your PPDP or individual PDPs?

Name of team member	Core skills and special interests	Specialist skills	Level of specialist skills				
			1	2	3	4	5

Health improvement plans

What are health improvement plans?

Health improvement plans (HImPs) are a way of expressing your identified health needs priorities, in order to determine what you wish to achieve.

Where do they fit?

These will then contribute to the primary-care group's 'Health Improvement Programme'. These programmes aim to improve the health of the local population.

An example and pro forma follow this page.

HEALTH IMPROVEMENT PLAN (HImP)

Aim	Objective	Start date	Benefit to patient	Outcome
Actively manage all our diabetes patients	Have an up-to-date diabetes register Review all diabetes patients at least once a year	January 2000 Ongoing	They receive up-to-date information on their condition Their glucose monitoring technique can be reviewed	Reduction in end-organ damage Later onset of complications
Improve the detection and subsequent management of depression	All clinical staff to increase their knowledge of the symptoms and management of depression	March 2000 and ongoing	Appropriate and timely therapeutic intervention	Reduction in suicide Reduction in consultations Fewer referrals
Actively manage post-MI patients	Prevent further MI occurring by prescribing aspirin and activity programmes	March 2000	Quality of life improved	Improve morbidity and mortality

HEALTH IMPROVEMENT PLAN (HImP)

Aim	Objective	Start date	Benefit to patient	Outcome

EFFECTIVE INTERVENTIONS

The next stage is to determine effective interventions as a specific of your HImP.

CLINICAL EFFECTIVENESS

Aim	Objective	Start date	Benefit to patient	Outcome
All diabetes patients have a glucose-monitoring meter	All patients accurately record their blood glucose	January 2000	Effective management of their condition	Reduction in complications and crises

PRACTICE DEVELOPMENT

Aim	Objective	Start date	Benefit to patient	Outcome
Up-to-date disease register	Review diabetes register	January 2000	All diabetes patients seen at least once a year	Accurate recall system in place for active management

EFFECTIVE INTERVENTIONS

The next stage is to determine effective interventions as a specific of your
HImP.

CLINICAL EFFECTIVENESS

Aim	Objective	Start date	Benefit to patient	Outcome

PRACTICE DEVELOPMENT

Aim	Objective	Start date	Benefit to patient	Outcome

Significant-event auditing

While looking at groups of patients can give GPs powerful insights into care, it can be difficult to turn discussion into action. It is common for repeat conventional audits to show little change for the better. However, we often dramatically change our behaviour when something happens to one patient, for example, a patient is registered partially sighted as a result of diabetic retinopathy, and we carry out fundoscopy with renewed enthusiasm.

Significant-event auditing is a method for harnessing the intellectual rigour of conventional audit to the emotional drive of 'adverse events'. It can therefore be:
- enjoyable (we all like discussing clinical cases);
- stimulating (it's *our* management of the patient that is being discussed!);
- evidence based (no wild decisions, but well-organized outcomes); and
- productive (decisions stick and care is improved).

The basic tenets

A group of significant cases is discussed, not only those where something has gone wrong, but also those that give insight into our care. The discussion is not intended to allocate blame, but to agree how, if at all, care can be improved. None of us is perfect and we need to learn from each other's imperfections. There are six possible outcomes from the discussion:

1 congratulations for care well given;
2 further investigation of the topic (search for evidence);
3 conventional audit;
4 immediate changes (only when justified);
5 identification of an educational need; and
6 decision that nothing needs to be done.

What is a significant event?

In short, it is anything that any member thinks notable, clinically or organizationally. Normally all MIs, infections, strokes, new cancers, unplanned pregnancies, attempted or successful suicides, osteoparotic fractures or acute visits for asthma, epilepsy or diabetes will be listed, as well as any patient complaint, administrative mix-up (visit requested but not carried out) or prescribing problem.

To maximize the success of introducing significant-event auditing into your practice, it is useful to think about the best ways to make the process appealing to the team. To be successful the participants must feel comfortable, both physically and professionally. This includes appropriate timing, maybe even with sandwiches for a working lunch. A no-blame culture needs to be adopted from the outset and this needs pointing out to all concerned. Some teams may find it more appealing to begin with just the doctors, adding other members of the team as confidence grows and the process develops.

Careful selection of the first event is essential. It is best to start with something that, while being important, is not too emotive; a very difficult or serious problem may fracture the team before enough confidence has been developed and the method is trusted. This will give the team the strength it will need to tackle more testing events in the future.

After nearly 10 years' experience of significant-event auditing, it is generally believed to be the single most powerful tool for improving care and identifying educational needs. For further details, it is recommended that you read *Occasional Paper 70* from the Royal College of General Practitioners (RCGP).

Ideas for subjects to use when thinking of significant events.

- New cancer cases.
- Unplanned pregnancies.
- Sudden death.
- Trauma, suicide.
- Drug reaction.
- Terminal care.
- Patient complaints.
- Breach of confidentiality.
- Aggressive patients.
- Home visits not carried out.
- Rota and staffing problems.
- Communication problems.
- Appointment problems.
- Legal—anything about this.
- Prescribing or dispensing error.

RECORDING A SIGNIFICANT EVENT (1)

	Action	Deadline
What happened? PG saw a Bath Hospital employee who wanted a termination but not at her own hospital		
How did it affect: **The patient** She wanted it to be carried out in Bristol to ensure confidentiality **You** Not sure how to go about referring Bath patients to Bristol **The practice** Also unsure about correct procedure for referral of patients to Bristol for termination of pregnancy		
Why did it happen? Not sure of the procedure/option		
Steps to be taken to avoid similar events in future: Contact British Pregnancy Advisory Service (BPAS) for details/Bristol consultants		
Learning needs revealed by the event: How to arrange termination out of the area for staff members, need efficient system to ensure patients are seen quickly	Dr A	5 January
How will these be met? Contact BPAS in Bristol for details of their service especially with regard to staff members		

RECORDING A SIGNIFICANT EVENT (1)

	Action	Deadline
What happened?		
How did it affect: **The patient** **You** **The practice**		
Why did it happen?		
Steps to be taken to avoid similar events in future:		
Learning needs revealed by the event:		
How will these be met?		

RECORDING A SIGNIFICANT EVENT (2)

Date of meeting: 31st January 2000

Events	Questions	Action
A. reported death of 66-year-old male patient with asthma and COPD—died suddenly at home		A. has done bereavement visit today—family extend thanks to all at the surgery
B. reported death of 96-year-old female—died of old age. Last seen 13 days ago	Any family?	No close relatives
C. has received notification of death in hospital of female patient. Coroner's report requested as she did not recover from anaesthetic after operation for fracture	Any family?	No immediate family known
C. raised problem of staff shortages in reception	How long and what needs to be done to help?	B. suggested district nurses could be asked to write out their prescription requests on blank scripts. All GPs to be given their own repeat requests on a daily basis to print themselves. H. to co-ordinate
A. reported new cancer. 56-year-old female seen by Sister X for breast examination. Known of lumps for a couple of months. Appointment made for last Thursday and scheduled for mastectomy at hospital today	How can we advise patients to present early?	A. to write an article for local paper B. to put article in newsletter C. to do notice-board in waiting room
C. reported on male patient following case conference today. Basically very suicidal but decision made not to section. <u>Beware</u> he has black belt in judo and a collection of knives and swords. Past history of alcohol abuse. Adamant he does not want to be sectioned and will defend himself. Has withdrawn all contact with mental health team		B. to notify Emergency Doctors Service
B. has had several patients recently who said they were not aware that they could see Dr F or Dr G instead of their registered GP	Should they be aware?	All patients were sent a letter clearly explaining the new system. Receptionists advise patients every day. B. to publicize in newsletter

RECORDING A SIGNIFICANT EVENT (2)

Date of meeting:

Events	Questions	Action

MINUTES OF SIGNIFICANT-EVENT AUDIT MEETING

Date:	1st February 2000
Present:	Dr A
	Dr B
	Dr C
	Practice nurse D
	Community nurses E & F
	Health visitor G
	Practice manager H
Apologies:	Partners I & J
	Practice nurses K & L

SIGNIFICANT EVENT NO. 1

Vaccination of minors

B.L., aged 13, came in for vaccinations with a relative. Unknown to the nurse, the relative left the surgery before the vaccination was completed

Outcome

Immediate change: the manager to instruct reception staff to always make sure if possible that a minor is never left in the surgery alone. If this happens they must inform the nurse in the surgery. Nurses to refuse to treat any minor if they know a relative is not present

SIGNIFICANT EVENT NO. 2

Routine review of sudden unexpected deaths within the last 3 months

7.15 a.m. Sunday. Male patient aged 53 years collapsed at home. Wife reported sudden onset of acute chest pain, pale, sweating. Ambulance attended—patient taken to hospital admitted Coronary Care Unit. Died Sunday p.m.—diagnosis acute anterior MI.

Discussion

Review of medical records. Patient registered with the practice 1994. Leaves wife aged 43 years and two children aged 10 and 13 years. Registration medical in 1996 incomplete. Known to be a smoker, BP 170/95, overweight at 107 kg advised to return for blood pressure check in 3 months. Last seen in February 1998 by locum and prescribed antibiotic for a chesty cough.

Following his death his widow said that his father also died suddenly of a heart attack in his early fifties and his brother had an MI in his forties. The patient has a number of risk factors for CHD and illustrates a potentially avoidable death

Possible interventions include:

1   A more thorough registration medical including taking a family history
2   Advice and support to stop smoking
3   Advice about diet and exercise
4   Monitoring and perhaps treatment of hypertension
5   Cholesterol screening

Outcome:

1   Audit to determine the percentage of patients who have not had a registration medical within 12 months of joining the practice
2   Re-design computer template to include weight, BMI, BP and smoking status, family history of CHD and stroke, cholesterol and advice about diet and exercise

Learning opportunities for PPDP and/or PDP

Practice to arrange an evening meeting to review the evidence of what is effective in the prevention of primary and secondary coronary heart disease

Using evidence in the management of common diseases

Evidence-based medicine (EBM) is the term used to describe the application of research evidence into everyday medical practice. Research can tell us which medical interventions really do work and which do not. Perhaps we are all guilty to a greater or lesser extent of practising medicine in a way that we have always done or we ignore evidence, e.g. prescribing antibiotics for viral infections. Most of us find it difficult to change the habits of a lifetime or are susceptible to patient pressure.

The aim of EBM is to ensure that clinical decisions are backed by the evidence of what is and what is not effective treatment, e.g. prescribing aspirin for the secondary prevention of coronary heart disease.

Reasons given for avoiding changing practice have been identified as scepticism, information overload and lack of time, skills, resources and motivation (Wilkinson *et al.* 1999). None of these could apply to you, could they?

Learning in groups

To help people make sense of evidence about effectiveness, the former Oxford Regional Health Authority set up the Critical Appraisal Skills Programme (CASP). In developing methods of helping people appraise reviews of evidence, CASP has worked closely with the UK Cochrane Centre and the McMaster University of Canada.

The CASP team, based in Oxford, holds training sessions and a number of Research & Development Support Unit Co-ordinators in the South & West region have learned to run workshops. The CASP team can be contacted by telephone on 01865 226968.

The workshop format is constantly evaluated and improved. There is a talk on clinical effectiveness including types of trials, reviews, and meta-analysis, together with some basic definitions of epidemiological and statistical terms. Participants then work in small groups to solve a problem scenario, such as whether or not dyspeptic patients who are positive for *Helicobacter pylori* should be treated with triple therapy. The problem is tackled by critically appraising an article about the clinical effectiveness of that problem.

Different participants will get different things from a CASP workshop. Some people only require an awareness of the importance of finding and appraising evidence, others will actually want to acquire the skills of critically appraising evidence, and a few will require the skills to enable them to write literature reviews.

Learning yourself

To find out which treatment works and which does not, you may wish to seek advice from your local medical librarian or you can look at the literature yourself.

The following list of publications may be helpful:
British Medical Journal
Lancet
British Journal of General Practice
Family Practice
Bandolier

MeReC Bulletins
Evidence Based Purchasing
Evidence Based Medicine
Journal of EBM
Drugs and Therapeutics Bulletin
University of York *Effective Health Care*

A list of useful websites can be found on page 175.

USING EVIDENCE IN THE MANAGEMENT OF COMMON DISEASES

Clinical problem

Secondary prevention of CHD

Is there any evidence about which treatment works and which does not?

Physical activity: British Regional Heart Study

Diet: recent British Heart Foundation information sheet for references

Stop smoking Aspirin: ISIS2 study

BP control: hypertension optimal treatment study

SMAC guidelines

4S study

How would I find out about the most effective treatment?

Medline and Cochrane databases

University of York's *Effective Health Care*

Guidelines publication

Drugs and Therapeutics Bulletin

USING EVIDENCE IN THE MANAGEMENT OF COMMON DISEASES

Use one sheet to discuss a problem

Clinical problem

Is there any evidence about which treatment works and which does not?

How would I find out about the most effective treatment?

Audit

There is now widespread recognition that a completed audit cycle is the educational vehicle for learning about change. For a variety of reasons, however, it can be very difficult to implement. A key issue is good preparation and a firm structure linked to a practical issue. A suggested format could be the following.

1 Define the precise area of care to be audited.
2 Prepare and plan involving all key members of the practice.
3 Review criteria defined and standards set.
4 Define a time for data collection.
5 Analyse data against the standards set.
6 Feed back data to the practice with agreement on change to be implemented and date for evaluation of change.

The crucial issue is that responsibility should be taken by an individual member of the practice (probably the manager) to oversee the audit within the practice. One suggestion is for the practice to develop an audit calendar for the year with specific areas being audited in specific months or quarters.

Example of an administrative audit

Title of audit

Registration of new-born babies in the practice.

Criterion

New-born babies in the practice should be registered within 6 weeks.

Standard set

Ninety-five per cent of babies will have completed registration forms by 6 weeks from birth.

Preparation and planning

The practice manager had been aware that the practice was missing out on new-born baby registrations because of the lack of a system for ensuring they were properly registered with the practice. He/she called a meeting of the partners, the health visitors and the practice nurse, and they decided to check the registration details over the last 6 months. The health visitor was delegated to collect the numbers of babies born in the practice over this time and the manager checked the date of birth and date of registration.

Data collection (1)

Thirty babies born with 20 registered at 6 weeks (66%).

Change to be implemented

A simple pro forma was drawn up with the headings: name of baby, date of birth and date registered. This was to be put in every patient's antenatal file and completed by the 6 week postnatal check.

Data collection (2)

This was carried out 6 months later. Forty babies born, 36 babies registered at six weeks (90%).

Conclusion

A simple tracking mechanism is usually necessary to ensure that patients do not fall through the system with consequent lack of follow-up and potential loss of income. New-born babies are often at risk of this, particularly in families where there are more pressures, such as the disadvantaged. A team effort and a tight protocol, simply kept, can ensure that these risks are minimized.

Example of a practice audit

A 65-year-old man arrives in the surgery with a proven bladder tumour. You note that microscopic haematuria had been recorded by the nurse 3 months previously but not followed up by the doctor, raising the possibility that the tumour could have been diagnosed earlier.

A significant-event analysis is carried out within the practice and it is further noted that there is no procedure for following up urine specimens sent to the laboratory. The practice decided that 95% of laboratory urine specimens should have a recorded follow-up in the records. A retrospective search through the case records over the past 4 weeks of laboratory urine specimens showed that 45% had a follow-up urine result in the records. All laboratory urine specimens were recorded in a book held by reception staff and a further column was added, which was then ticked when the follow-up sample was recorded. Gaps could then be easily identified and followed up. Three months later a repeat collection of data over a similar period was carried out and the percentage of laboratory urine specimens followed up had risen to 88%.

Lessons learned were that a simple change in the recording method allowed easy follow-up and, in particular, identification of defaulters. Costs were saved by defining those specimens samples which should be tested in the practice and those which should be sent to a laboratory. Sub-optimal care was rectified by improved follow-up and management.

After reading the above audits you may wish to tick the box if you felt that the criterion was present.

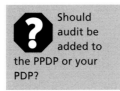

Should audit be added to the PPDP or your PDP?

Criteria		Present
Reason for choice of audit	Potential for change relevant for the unit/ general practice	❏
Criterion/criteria chosen	Relevant to audit subject and justifiable (e.g. current literature)	❏
Standards set	Set targets towards a standard with a suitable timescale	❏
Preparation and planning	Evidence of teamwork and adequate discussion where appropriate	❏
Data collection (1)	Results compared against standard	❏
Change(s) to be evaluated	Example supplied	❏
Data collection (2)	Comparison with data collection (1) and standard	❏
Conclusions	Summary of main issues (e.g. bullet points)	❏

Using complaints to improve practice

Nobody likes to receive a complaint about their practice. They cause a lot of heartache amongst the team and are time consuming.

Each practice should at this stage have evolved their own practice-based complaints procedure. Currently the emphasis is on resolution of problems, where possible, in-house. Most complaints can be resolved in this way but some may go further and even involve litigation or the use of the formal NHS (1996) procedures.

The aim of a complaints system should be to satisfy the needs of the complainants. Often this may only need an adequate explanation and apology where appropriate, whilst being fair to all concerned. Honesty, courtesy and sympathy in the handling of a complaint will often go a long way towards defusing a potentially difficult situation.

Practices have a duty to deal with complaints quickly and sensitively and to keep written records of all contacts with patients. Patients must also be made aware of their rights to take their complaint to the relevant health authority. Written information about the complaints procedure should be available to patients in the surgery.

Each practice should nominate an administrative member of staff and a doctor to deal with complaints. Meticulous record keeping is of paramount importance. Copies of letters must be kept and notes, dates and times of all telephone conversations should be logged.

If a patient complains in person, say at reception, then the receptionist should offer an immediate meeting with a member of staff in private, so that the complaint can be recorded on an in-house complaint form. This should be completed, dated, timed and signed by the patient and the member of staff. The patient can be given information about the complaint procedure there and then.

All complaints should be reviewed regularly and you should try to categorize them. By so doing, you may be able to identify deficiencies within the practice, both clinical and non-clinical, which if addressed promptly and honestly can improve the quality of the service that you can provide. Analysis of complaints fits in well with the process of significant-event auditing as described on page 60.

> **!** Use each complaint as potential for learning
> Look at what has been learnt from the complaint

Learning from complaints

Complaints to the practice can be a valuable tool to look at your practice, how it works and how staff perform within the team. Complaints seem to involve mainly appointment systems, telephone answering delays, prescriptions and staff attitudes as the major grievances.

Consider the following example

The practice operates a twice-daily emergency surgery using a triage nurse and also a routine appointment system. One doctor is designated the duty doctor from 8 a.m. to 7 p.m. and sees all emergency patients and does all emergency visits. The remaining partners have booked surgeries at varying times during the day. Out of hours is covered by a co-operative.

A patient found it difficult to get an appointment as a bank holiday approached, and went to the Primary Care Emergency Centre for advice. She then had to get an appointment at the practice but had to wait 5 days to do so. She complained that she could not be seen sooner and criticized the system. Her own doctor was on leave at that time.

? Do we need to do anything as a result?
If we do, what needs doing and how should it be done?
Should this be added to the PPDP?

The practice manager dealt with the problem by letter. The manager's reply pointed out, after an apology, that:

1 the existence of a same-day service for urgent cases;
2 other doctors covered for absent colleagues; and
3 there was a facility for assessment or advice from a triage nurse.

Nothing further was heard. The learning points were:

• Despite publicity, the surgery systems were not widely known.
• The receptionists needed more training to help patients who were confused about the new system.
• Publicizing the surgery systems (at regular intervals), would be useful.
• Handling the complaint promptly and courteously appeared to have resolved the problem satisfactorily.

Complaints procedure

The following flowchart may be of help.

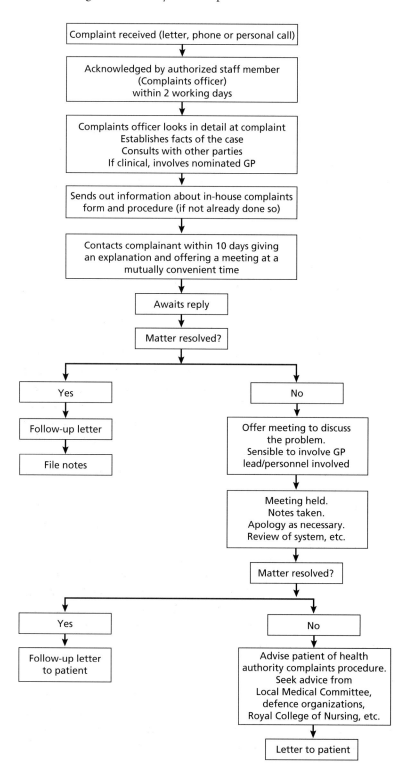

You and your practice

The primary-care group

Whilst your team is developing its practice plan using this workbook, it is already part of a larger organization: the primary-care group (PCG). Your PCG will have its own structures for developing quality and showing good practice through clinical governance and (with other local organizations) the health improvement plan (HImP). Your practice and PCG can both benefit from good communication and sharing of information.

To do this you need:
- a PPDP;
- an active clinical governance group in your PCG;
- a clearly identified clinical governance lead in your practice attending the group; and
- good communication between clinical governance leads and the partnership board for the health improvement plan.

Clinical governance is a new name for established concepts of quality of care. It provides a framework for better care through personal and team development, and sharing best practice. It involves identifying team members' needs and helping to achieve them. It is thus closely allied with the concepts behind this workbook. Local primary-care tutors will work to provide educational opportunities to meet the needs identified in PPDPs and clinical governance groups. Eventually each PCG will have its own educational support from a tutor, a facilitator and others, and will develop as an educational unit.

Both clinical governance and health improvement planning are activities which need grass roots input as well as national frameworks: 'bottom up' as well as 'top down'.

The health needs assessment and clinical audit activities within your practice development will provide this vital 'grass roots' information.

Everyone involved can call for advice and assistance from GP and nurse tutors, GP trainers and other facilitators. Links with the regional educational structures will be valuable as a source of expertise, personnel and educational training opportunities.

Example

Your practice needs assessment has identified substance misuse as a local problem. Substance misusers play GPs and practices against one another, and the response is inconsistent. You perceive a need to examine this problem and report this to the clinical governance group via your practice clinical governance lead.

The local GP tutor responds to this educational need and convenes a study workshop to examine the best way of dealing with this in the local area. The workshop reports its conclusions to the PCG. The clinical governance group gathers information from all local practices about scale and range of problems. The PCG responds with a local management plan and guidelines, and reports to the partnership board, which then includes a section on substance misuse in the HImP.

With resources targeted to this problem, GPs are assisted by substance misuse advisers and start to address the problem in a consistent and effective way.

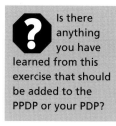

Is there anything you have learned from this exercise that should be added to the PPDP or your PDP?

Referral data

Completing the table on the following page should help you to understand how your own clinical practice compares with the average for your area.

This comparison will not give you answers, nor determine whether your practice is right or wrong. It will help you to highlight clinical areas where there is significant variation from the average (+/- 20% would be a useful starting point). You should be able to obtain this information from your health authority (Public Health), PCG or local district general hospital.

Following this analysis you may wish to seek guidance in understanding significant variations in order to inform future clinical practice.

Practice population profile

Total	Gender	0–4	5–15	16–44	45–64	65–74	75–84	85+	Expected births
	Male								
	Female								

Do you want to compare this profile to 1 year ago and 5 years ago?

Referrals for year ending
(exclude private referrals)

A Speciality	B Number	C Number per 1000 population	D Health authority average per 1000 population	E Percentage variation from average
General surgery				
Urology				
Orthopaedic				
ENT				
Ophthalmology				
Oral surgery				
Neurosurgery				
Plastic surgery				
Pain clinic				
General medical				
Gastrology				
Direct access—Endoscopy				
Direct access—Colonoscopy				
Haematology				
Audiology				
Cardiology				
Dermatology				
Thoracic				
Nephrology				
Medical oncology				
Neurology				
Rheumatology				
Paediatrics				
Geriatrics				
Mental illness				
Child & adolescent psychiatry				
Psychotherapy				
All other				
Radiology—X-ray referrals				
Physiotherapy—All referrals				
Pathology—All requests				
Total				

continued on p. 80

A Speciality	B Number	C Number per 1000 population	D Health authority average per 1000 population	E Percentage variation from average
Emergency admissions				
Surgery				
Medicine				
Paediatrics				
Geriatrics				

Note: You may need to use only relevant population to complete column C & D.

e.g. Paediatrics 0–15 population, Geriatrics 65 ± population.

PACT prescribing

Every GP is provided on a quarterly basis with detailed information about their prescribing by the Prescription Pricing Authority (PPA). Non-principals working regularly within a practice can collect PACT data by placing a red 'D' on the prescription. This is powerful information and enables us to compare our performance against our colleagues both locally and nationally. It also gives us information about our prescribing in British National Formulary (BNF) Therapeutic Groups and a list of our most expensive prescriptions. It gives us the opportunity to look critically and monitor our prescribing and perhaps institute changes, which can be formally adopted by the whole practice and written into the PPDP.

An example and pro forma to help you to use prescribing information to inform future prescribing patterns can be found on page 82.

THE PRACTICE PRESCRIBING COSTS FOR THE LAST QUARTER

Were above/~~below~~ the health authority equivalent by	↑ 7%
Were above/~~below~~ the national equivalent by	↑ 5%

BNF therapeutic group significantly above/below health authority equivalent
Significantly above in antibiotics, CVS and CNS

The ten most expensive drugs used in the practice are:

1 Zestril

2 Losec

3 Seroxat

4 Colostomy bags

5 Pulmicort

6 Zocor

7 Augmentin

8 Atorvastatin

9 Diclofenac

10 Losartan

The practice generic prescribing rate is ~~above~~/below the health authority equivalent by	↑ 20%
~~Above~~/below the national equivalent by	↑ 10%
The practice generic prescribing rate is	30%
Has there been any significant change in the practice's PACT figures over the last 12 months	YES ☑ NO ☐
If YES why has this change taken place?	
Increased generic prescribing rate by 5% and reduction in costs from 10% above health authority equivalent to 7%	
Do you plan to use this prescribing information to inform your PPDP?	YES ☑ NO ☐
If YES, how?	
1 To increase generic prescribing 2 To introduce a practice formulary	

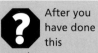

After you have done this exercise:

• Do you plan to use this prescribing information to inform your PPDP?

• If YES, how?

THE PRACTICE PRESCRIBING COSTS FOR THE LAST QUARTER

Were above/below the health authority equivalent by	
Were above/below the national equivalent by	

BNF therapeutic group significantly above/below health authority equivalent

The ten most expensive drugs used in the practice are:

1

2

3

4

5

6

7

8

9

10

The practice generic prescribing rate is above/below the health authority equivalent by	
Above/below the national equivalent by	
The practice generic prescribing rate is	
Has there been any significant change in the practice's PACT figures over the last 12 months	YES ❑ NO ❑
If YES why has this change taken place?	
Do you plan to use this prescribing information to inform your PPDP?	YES ❑ NO ❑
If YES, how?	

Performance indicators in primary care

The following is an example of a typical box plot that the health authority might publish as a performance indicator (PI) to measure asthma care in practice.

The percentage of patients in a practice (>15 years old) who have a diagnosis of asthma:

Minimum   **Maximum 15%**

X

Your practice

What does this PI tell you about this practice's diagnosis or management of asthma? How might you use this information to improve this practice's care of asthmatics?

What is its relevance?

• The PI does not tell us anything about the clinical care of asthmatic patients. Perhaps the practice does not have any agreed protocols or policies. Perhaps there is no formalized disease register in place.

• On the other hand, the practice's prescribing of inhaled steroids and beta-antagonists is well above the PCG and county average. How can this be if we do not have the patients to treat? Do we have a lot of patients with COPD? Does our prescribing need to be looked at or is there simply a problem with recording the information?

• Maybe the practice should be looking to improve the care of asthmatics from this position of relative ignorance. Perhaps it would be worth considering a dedicated asthma clinic. How do you set this up? Who will run it? Are all the nurses trained? How do we organize call and re-call systems for the patients?

• Should the practice operate a disease register? Will this be computer or paper based? Who will run it? How will it be kept up to date? If it is computer based, how will you get all the partners and nurses to use it consistently with similar codes?

• You remember reading something about an audit some time ago. It was to do with assuming that if the data are not available, then it has probably not been carried out. Maybe we ought to adopt an attitude of 'We used to think we knew what we were doing, but now we really do know—because we checked'.

• You can obtain details from your health authority or PCG on how your practice performance compares to other practices, e.g. percentage of inadequate cervical smears.

How might PIs be used to identify learning needs?

Performance indicators might be produced to demonstrate how one organization is performing or how that organization compares with another. The organization might be a health authority, PCG or practice, or indeed an individual GP.

The information we have returned to the health authority as part of our statutory (Red Book) reporting for chronic disease management for asthma shows that we have fewer asthma patients than most other practices.
Is this because
• We have not sent the correct information?
• We have sent it but the health authority has incorrectly recorded it?
• We do not have a systematic system for recording the diagnosis to enable accurate reporting?

1 What do you think is the purpose of PIs?

2 What are the advantages and disadvantages of commonly used PIs? (HINT! Are PIs useful in simply informing or comparing?)

3 Do they bring about a change in behaviour? How do they achieve this?

4 Do most of them measure the most useful and relevant things to you—as a clinician—and your practice? If not, how might PIs be changed to measure something more useful?

5 How might PIs be improved?

6 Which of the currently available PIs do you think are relevant to bringing about a change in clinical behaviour?

7 Why did you identify these PIs and not others?

Research and development

Research is exciting and rewarding, and is fundamental to the health sciences. Historically, the epidemiological research undertaken by GPs has made a significant contribution to the health of the nation, for example: the aetiology and eradication of smallpox; the causes of yellow fever and typhoid fever; the epidemiology of heart disease; and the spread of infection in infectious hepatitis.

Interested and enthusiastic individual practitioners can do important research. However, some research questions are difficult to answer by one GP on his/her own, and may require a much larger population base than that within one practice. A team approach, with the active involvement of a number of participating practices, opens up more research opportunities and the potential for the pooling of expertise. One way of linking with other GPs with research interests is through the Primary Care Research Networks (PCRN).

Although most NHS contacts occur and end in general practice, currently only a small proportion of clinical research involves general practice. There are many reasons for this, not least the lack of time and space in most surgeries. However, other barriers, such as the lack of availability of research training, academic support, and research funding, can now be overcome. The research networks can provide help and information. The NHS Executive provides expert advice and assistance to all healthcare professionals on the design and conduct of R&D projects, in both the primary and secondary care sectors.

Perhaps you are not so keen on undertaking or participating in original research, but are concerned that your healthcare decisions should be based on best research evidence, not opinion or guesswork! There are courses which focus on the sources of evidence and how to find them, as well as on how to critically appraise research findings. The research networks can provide you with appropriate information.

Undertaking research, finding relevant literature, and appraising it are only part of the process of evidence-based practice. The other two components relate to deriving the important questions in the first place and, at the other extreme, applying the results.

As far as the former is concerned, questions are most often initiated within a specific patient encounter. Please let the research community know where the gaps in research are and what should be the priorities for further research. Calls for applications for research funding in these areas are then likely to be initiated.

Finally, GPs make important healthcare decisions within the unique patient–practitioner consultation. This points to the importance of practitioners being up to date and knowing what is best evidence. Please take advantage of some of the help which is available. You will then have the flexibility to use the evidence within the patient consultation, taking into account the situation and preferences of a specific patient.

- Are you a member of a primary-care research network?
- Do you want to learn more about R&D methods?
- Have you identified any important research questions in your practice?
- Are you or your practice thinking about getting involved with research?
- Is this something you should put in your PPDP or your PDP?

Staff appraisals

General practice relies heavily on staff to contribute fully to the smooth running of the organization not only as a provider of healthcare but as a business. The GP has to be familiar with the concept of performance management, which involves managing the business of general practice for today and to develop it for the future. He/she needs to be assured that all members of the PHCT:

1 do what the organization needs them to do;
2 are willing to improve their personal contribution to the organization; and
3 want to improve the overall performance of the organization.

Each member of the PHCT should have a clearly defined role within the team and this should be backed up by a written, mutually agreed, contract, setting out all the terms and conditions of their job. All staff should have a clear idea of their responsibilities within the team and to whom they can turn for advice.

To monitor, evaluate and improve performance of his/her staff, the GP needs to be familiar with the process of appraisal. The essential process of appraisal is one of mutual trust and co-operation, it is not meant to be a stick with which to beat employees, but rather a structured discussion looking at the employee's current performance and future aspirations.

The GP will have to decide how the appraisal process should be implemented and who should appraise whom. (There are numerous publications available and help can be obtained from your health authority.)

In essence, a good appraisal system should include the following features.
• Enable staff to be clear about their role within the organization.
• Enable staff to be aware of the responsibilities of their current position within the practice.
• Enable staff to be aware of the minimum standards expected of them.
• Enable staff to be aware of the lines of management within the practice.
• Provide the opportunity for a frank discussion about personal performance, future aspirations and ways and means of rewarding good performance.
• Give an opportunity to plan for future career developments: address areas of concern, etc., all within an agreed timescale and a review of these plans.
• Appraisals are designed to get the best from employees and are a regular event.

The appraisal interview

There must be a formal structure to the whole process and the appraisal should be arranged so as to allow an unhurried and useful discussion with the employee.

Who should do the appraising?

This needs to be decided after discussion; the appraisal can either be conducted by the practice manager, or the practice manager and the GP with responsibility for staff.

The process

• The employee should complete a **pre-appraisal checklist** (see p. 90) so as to be ready for the interview. Modesty is a common trait and should be recognized. The questionnaire should be completed honestly and used as a basis for discussion at the interview.

• The interview should draw on points raised in the pre-appraisal checklist and fully discuss the results, followed by completing an *assessment of performance form* (see p. 94).

• Finally there should be a summary of the appraisal and a personal action plan drawn up (see p. 98).

• A review process of the Personal Action Plan should be agreed with the employee ensuring that no empty promises are made.

Finally, both the appraisee and appraiser might find the *learning points from the appraisal* form (see p. 100) helpful.

The practice manager is ideally placed to manage the process and the review system, and provide any follow-up, monitoring and support to the employee as required.

PRE-APPRAISAL CHECKLIST

It will soon be time for the annual appraisal of your performance in your job with us. To save time and to ensure that we talk about you and your job, please look at the questions given below. Try to answer them by yourself as honestly as possible and do not be modest.

These questions and your answers will form the basis of the appraisal interview and are designed to help you build on your own strengths and offer opportunities in the future to do so.

---

1 What is your job?

Treatment room nurse

---

2 Does your job description need updating/changing?

Yes

---

3 Indicate how good you think you are in dealing with the following areas of activity:

	Excellent	V. Good	Good	Moderate
Knowledge of job		✓		
Ability to organize			✓	
Solving problems			✓	
Making decisions	✓			
Relationships with colleagues		✓		
Relationships with patients		✓		
Ability to communicate			✓	
Handling paperwork				✓
Verbal manner on phone and face to face		✓		

---

4 Have you had any noteworthy accomplishments, which your manager should be aware of? (awards, exams, etc.)

Asthma Diploma

Infection control certificate

---

5 What should your aims and objectives be for the next year?

Set up practice triage

Review existing asthma systems with practice manager

---

6 What training or help do you require to attain these objectives?

Triage nurse training

Admin support for nurses

7 What are your career aims?

To become nurse practitioner

8 What particular parts of the job interest you?

To become a more independent practitioner working → EBM–common diseases

9 What particular parts interest you least?

Administration

10 Are there any other matters you would like to discuss with your manager? Now is your chance!

Job description

Funding for training

PRE-APPRAISAL CHECKLIST

It will soon be time for the annual appraisal of your performance in your job with us. To save time and to ensure that we talk about you and your job, please look at the questions given below. Try to answer them by yourself as honestly as possible and do not be modest.

These questions and your answers will form the basis of the appraisal interview and are designed to help you build on your own strengths and offer opportunities in the future to do so.

1 What is your job?

2 Does your job description need updating/changing?

3 Indicate how good you think you are in dealing with the following areas of activity:

	Excellent	V. Good	Good	Moderate
Knowledge of job				
Ability to organize				
Solving problems				
Making decisions				
Relationships with colleagues				
Relationships with patients				
Ability to communicate				
Handling paperwork				
Verbal manner on phone and face to face				

4 Have you had any noteworthy accomplishments, which your manager should be aware of? (awards, exams, etc.)

5 What should your aims and objectives be for the next year?

6 What training or help do you require to attain these objectives?

7 What are your career aims?

8 What particular parts of the job interest you?

9 What particular parts interest you least?

10 Are there any other matters you would like to discuss with your manager? Now is your chance!

ASSESSMENT OF PERFORMANCE

Name: F Nightingale

Date: 1/2/2000

Knowledge of work

- Knowledge and understanding of own job/knowledge of procedures, rules, etc.
- Knowledge and understanding of how her job relates to that of others

Comments

We have agreed that Flo will become adept at organizing and demonstrating her skills at clinical audit with administrative support

Doing the job

- Ability to understand and assimilate information
- Ability to apply knowledge in a practical situation. To take sensible and practical action. Set priorities and where necessary seek advice
- Use of initiative. Suggests improvements. Finds out all relevant information and acts promptly

Comments

Flo is keen to develop her role as nurse practitioner and the practice is keen to introduce a triage system and will support her training in this

Approach to work

- Self-reliance and responsibility (can be left to organize and complete a job without supervision)
- Method of working (accuracy, thoroughness, methodical and systematic)
- Performance under pressure (self-controlled, able to be resilient and adaptable)

Comments

Admin skills need developing along with IT skills and expertise which will release pressure of workload
Practice manager to give advice on systematic approach.

Relationships with colleagues, patients and doctors

- Verbal communication skills—able to express ideas and information clearly and concisely
- Working relations with others (ability to work within the team in a helpful, co-operative, tactful manner)
- Patient relations (pleasant, informed, helpful and confident when dealing with patients?)

Comments

Needs to develop team rapport with subordinates

ASSESSMENT OF PERFORMANCE

Name:

Date:

Knowledge of work

Comments

Doing the job

Comments

Approach to work

Comments

Relationships with colleagues, patients and doctors

Comments

PERSONAL ACTION PLAN FOR 1999/2000

Name: F Nightingale

Date: September 1999

Knowledge of work

Flo has a good working knowledge of her subject and within 12 months will work towards the role of nurse practitioner and her progress will be reviewed in 6/12 months

Doing the job

Administration of treatment room will be improved by increased administrative support (stat) and improving systems. Clinical audit will automatically follow and this will be reviewed in 12 months

Future plans? (include career plans, training needs, etc.)

Flo will attend nurse triage training organized by the health authority in January 2000 and a training course on administration for senior treatment room nurses in April 2000

PERSONAL ACTION PLAN FOR 1999/2000

Name:	Date:

Knowledge of work

Doing the job

Future plans? (include career plans, training needs, etc.)

LEARNING POINTS FROM THE APPRAISAL

What went well?

Appreciation

Enlightening

What went badly?

Threatening

Enlightening

Could it have been done better?

More practice manager involvement

If so, how?

Completion of forms and attendance at review

LEARNING POINTS FROM THE APPRAISAL

What went well?

What went badly?

Could it have been done better?

If so, how?

Partner review system

The partner review process is designed to enhance the overall performance of the practice by providing supportive and constructive feedback to each individual partner on aspects of their performance. The outcome of the review can link into each doctor's personal development plan (PDP).

Procedure

The plan is for each partner within the practice to complete a review once a year. In a four-partner practice this could be divided into one review every quarter. The review needs to be carried out with the help of another partner acting as a mentor or facilitator. It is the role of the partner acting as the mentor to ensure that the review is appropriate and that feedback is suitably and sufficiently explored. Do not forget to include regular non-principals working within the practice.

For this process to be successful the partner being reviewed should be free to nominate his/her own mentor. The whole process needs to be conducted in a 'no blame' environment with the emphasis being on constructive feedback to facilitate positive development.

The role of the facilitating partner is to ensure that feedback is fair and balanced, and that the feedback is sufficiently explored and discussed to the satisfaction of the partner being reviewed.

The documentation to support the review process includes the following.

1 **Partner Review Feedback Form** (see p. 104). To be completed by all partners individually (and the practice manager) and the partner being reviewed—to be discussed at the assessment interview.

2 **Partner Review Summary Record of Discussion** (see p. 108). To be completed by the partner facilitating the review, either during the review or immediately upon completion, and passed to the partner being reviewed.

3 **Plan for Continued Professional and Personal Development** (see p. 110). To be completed by the partner being reviewed within 7 days of the review and returned to the facilitating partner.

One copy of all documents to be kept in the partner's file. The practice manager may wish to manage the process and the review system, and provide any follow-up, monitoring and support to the partners as required.

PARTNER REVIEW FEEDBACK FORM

To:	From:
Date:	**Date of review:**

1 What do you particularly value about this partner's input to the successful operation and development of the practice?

(a) In terms of their clinical practice?

Enthusiastic over clinical challenge

Keeps well up to date and always seeks further opinion

(b) In terms of their contribution to business planning and development of the image of the practice?

Innovative tenacious approach

Can lose focus

(c) In terms of their personal qualities and knowledge?

Dynamic

Enjoys new ideas

2 What has this partner particularly achieved over the last year, which is worthy of note?

Co-ordinating Investors in People

Winding down fundholding

Staff appraisal

Started regular column for local press

3 Strengths and weaknesses
Please identify strengths and weakness against the following criteria:
S = Strength   W = Weakness   SS = Clear strength   WW = Clear weakness

	Strength or weakness	Comments
Patient satisfaction		
Relationships with patients	SS	
Keeping to appointment times	S	
Timely and appropriate referral	S	
Staff satisfaction		
Operational communication	S/W	Volatile
Administrative efficiency	S	
Approachable style	SS	
Development of knowledge in others	SS	
Contribution to partnership		
Good ideas	S	
Critical evaluation	S	
Keeping things on track	S/W	Takes too much on
Getting things done	S/W	
External liaison	SS	
Contribution to profit		
Timely completion of claims	S	
Perception of the practice by the wider world	SS	
Financial control	S	
Clinical efficiency	S	

4 In what ways do you think the practice or individual partners could give more support to this person?

Ensure does not take on too much

Decrease list size to support other projects

Forced to take half day

5 Any other issues which you would like to discuss at the review

Clinical data for new computer timescales

Signed: **Date:**

PARTNER REVIEW FEEDBACK FORM

To:	From:
Date:	**Date of review:**

1 What do you particularly value about this partner's input to the successful operation and development of the practice?

(a) In terms of their clinical practice?

(b) In terms of their contribution to business planning and development of the image of the practice?

(c) In terms of their personal qualities and knowledge?

2 What has this partner particularly achieved over the last year, which is worthy of note?

3 Strengths and weaknesses
Please identify strengths and weakness against the following criteria:
S = Strength   W = Weakness   SS = Clear strength   WW = Clear weakness

	Strength or weakness	Comments
Patient satisfaction		
Relationships with patients		
Keeping to appointment times		
Timely and appropriate referral		
Staff satisfaction		
Operational communication		
Administrative efficiency		
Approachable style		
Development of knowledge in others		
Contribution to partnership		
Good ideas		
Critical evaluation		
Keeping things on track		
Getting things done		
External liaison		
Contribution to profit		
Timely completion of claims		
Perception of the practice by the wider world		
Financial control		
Clinical efficiency		

4 In what ways do you think the practice or individual partners could give more support to this person?

5 Any other issues which you would like to discuss at the review

Signed:	Date:

PARTNER REVIEW SUMMARY RECORD OF DISCUSSION

Name:

Summary of specific achievements over the last year

Co-ordinating Investors in People

Winding down fundholding

Staff appraisal

Started regular column for local press

Strengths and weaknesses

(a) Strengths

Relationships with patients

Approachable and keen to develop others

External liaison

Perception of the practice by the wider world

(b) Weaknesses

Takes on too much and at times unable to keep on track and can lose focus

PARTNER REVIEW SUMMARY RECORD OF DISCUSSION

Name:

Summary of specific achievements over the last year

Strengths and weaknesses

(a) Strengths

(b) Weaknesses

PLAN FOR CONTINUED PROFESSIONAL AND PERSONAL DEVELOPMENT

Name:

1 Professional development	Timescale	Resources required/ measure of your success
Clinical practice **Your objectives?** Audit appropriateness of my referrals	12 months	Clinical data PACT data Consultant feedback
Clinical knowledge **Your objectives?** MBA	5 years	Finance Internet Journals Partners' support University
Other vocational development **Your objectives?** See above Teaching qualification	2 years	Finance Practice support Time
Clinical efficiency and use of resources **Your objectives?** Work within guidelines/protocols laid down by PCG	12 months	Good communication with PCG

2 Personal and management skills	Timescale	Resources required/measure of your success
Contribution to patient satisfaction **Your objectives?** Timely appointment system	Ongoing	Audits
Contribution to staff satisfaction **Your objectives?** Be more amenable and not so hot-headed	STAT	Propranolol
Contribution to the team **Your objectives?** Clinical governance-led PCG	2 years	Practice support Time
Contribution to profit and the development of the practice **Your objectives?** Timely/appropriate information for claims	STAT	New computer system (reduce duplication)
Personal management skills **Your objectives?** Work with new practice manager —induction	STAT	Partner support Time

Signed:	Date:

PLAN FOR CONTINUED PROFESSIONAL AND PERSONAL DEVELOPMENT

Name:

1 Professional development	Timescale	Resources required/ measure of your success
Clinical practice **Your objectives?**		
Clinical knowledge **Your objectives?**		
Other vocational development **Your objectives?**		
Clinical efficiency and use of resources **Your objectives?**		

2 Personal and management skills	Timescale	Resources required/measure of your success
Contribution to patient satisfaction **Your objectives?**		
Contribution to staff satisfaction **Your objectives?**		
Contribution to the team **Your objectives?**		
Contribution to profit and the development of the practice **Your objectives?**		
Personal management skills **Your objectives?**		

Signed:	Date:

The practice professional development plan

The practice professional development plan (PPDP) is the central document by which the practice collates information about its activity and aspirations. The main *purpose* of the plan is to enable the practice and primary healthcare team (PHCT) to focus on the objectives and priorities for future years and to identify continuing needs.

The PPDP is first and foremost for the practice and the *process* of producing the plan is as important as the final document. The production of the plan should involve all PHCT members.

The headings discussed in this workbook are given below as part of the review process, but there will, of course, be other subjects which are not covered, such as premises, co-operatives.

The plan will form an important *link* with the primary-care group (PCG) and ensures that it is aware of your plans and development needs. It will also enable you to demonstrate your achievements in line with national and local priorities.

Components of the plan
- Mission statement

Example

> Our aim is to provide a comprehensive, friendly, professional and personal service, with time to discuss our patients' healthcare concerns. We endeavour to make it easy for our patients to make an appointment to see their doctor, nurse or other healthcare professional. We intend to be part of our local community and a centre for excellence in the provision of primary healthcare, with in-house provision of a range of medical services. We will provide this service by maintaining an efficient and profitable business.

- Review of previous year's objectives (no example)
- Health needs assessment (p. 19)
  Creating a profile of your practice population (p. 20)
  Key features of your practice population (p. 22)
  Identification of top health problems in your practice (p. 24)
  Prioritizing the list (p. 28)
  Planning interventions (p. 30)
  Creating an action plan (p. 34)
  New priorities (p. 36)
- The primary healthcare team (p. 38)
- Skill mix of the primary healthcare team (p. 47)
- Health improvement plans (p. 55)
- Significant-event auditing (p. 60)
  Using evidence in the management of common diseases (p. 68)
  Audit (p. 72)
  Using complaints to improve practice (p. 74)

❗ The list on pages 114–115 is a template of the sections in this book. Use it to bring forward anything from the individual sections which you have identified as being suitable to add to your PPDP.

- You and your practice (p. 77)
  Referral data (p. 78)
  PACT—prescribing (p. 81)
  Performance indicators in primary care (p. 84)
  Research and development (p. 86)
- Staff appraisals (p. 87)
- Partner review system (p. 103)
- The practice professional development plan (p. 114)

PRACTICE PROFESSIONAL DEVELOPMENT PLAN

Review each section of this book	What are the key things we have identified?	Practice objectives to be added to PPDP	How are we going to do this? (optional)
Health needs assessment	• Elderly list • High instance of chronic disease	Improve management of chronic disease	
Creating a profile of the practice population	Predominantly middle class—some rural poverty		
Key features of the practice population	20% practice pop > 65 yr		
Identification of top health problems in your practice	1 CHD 2 COAD 3 Hypertension 4 Diabetes mellitus	1 CHD 2 COAD 3 Hypertension 4 Diabetes mellitus	Use PMS pilot status to improve quality assurance
Prioritizing the list	As above	As above	
Planning interventions	Poor quality assurance in the management of chronic disease	Improve the management of chronic disease	Run base-line audits and develop recall system
Creating an action plan	Involve the whole PHCT		
New priorities	Roll out improved management of chronic disease to all age groups		
The primary healthcare team	Poor integration of nursing and social services	Development of integrated nursing team and appointment of link worker	Start with practice away day
Skill mix of the primary healthcare team	Experienced nurses, interested in EBM and research		
Health improvement plans Clinical effectiveness	Improve management of CHD Prevention of CHD	Improve management of CHD Start with secondary prevention of CHD	Redesign evidence-based computer templates

Review each section of this book	What are the key things we have identified?	Practice objectives to be added to PPDP	How are we going to do this? (optional)
Significant-event auditing	Less than optimum management of CHD	Prioritize management of CHD	
Using evidence in the management of common diseases	Start with CHD	As above	
Audit	Problem with read-codes for diagnosis of asthma and protocol for accuracy of data entry	Improve in-house management of asthma	
Using complaints to improve practice	Poor perception by patients of telephone answering and patient relations	Improve customer relations	Customer relations training for reception staff
You and your practice			
Referral data	Higher than average referral rates dermatology and ENT, high emergency admission rates	To reduce referral and acute admissions to below local average	Individual PDPs and to understand why referral rates/admissions are high
PACT—Prescribing	Low generic prescribers	Develop and agree practice formulary	
Performance indicators in primary care	Above average inadequate smear rate	To reduce to below local average	Multi-disciplinary workshop for all clinical staff, review clinical skills
Research and development	Special interest to nurses	To develop an EBM and research culture in the practice	Training for nurses in EBM, CASP and research methods
Staff appraisals	Reception staff lack knowledge of PCGs and organization/changes in NHS	To Investors of People award	Offer individual training to reception staff
Partner review system	One partner x2 average referral in dermatology One partner x3 average referral in ENT	To reduce referral to below local average	Add dermatology and ENT updates to individual partner's PDPs

PRACTICE PROFESSIONAL DEVELOPMENT PLAN

Review each section of this book	What are the key things we have identified?	Practice objectives to be added to PPDP	How are we going to do this? (optional)
Health needs assessment			
Creating a profile of the practice population			
Key features of the practice population			
Identification of top health problems in your practice			
Prioritizing the list			
Planning interventions			
Creating an action plan			
New priorities			
The primary healthcare team			
Skill mix of the primary healthcare team			
Health improvement plans Clinical effectiveness			

Review each section of this book	What are the key things we have identified?	Practice objectives to be added to PPDP	How are we going to do this? (optional)
Significant-event auditing			
Using evidence in the management of common diseases			
Audit			
Using complaints to improve practice			
You and your practice			
Referral data			
PACT—Prescribing			
Performance indicators in primary care			
Research and development			
Staff appraisals			
Partner review system			

OBJECTIVES OF THE PRACTICE

Why was this chosen?	What are we going to do?	How will this benefit our patients?	Do we require any additional resources?	How will we know that we have been successful?	Any need for further training?	Priority	Outcome (clinical audit against key markers)
• Health needs assessment exercise • Elderly list • Health improvement plan (HImP) • Good evidence of clinical effectiveness	• Base-line audit • Enter data in evidence-based computer template • Develop a recall system	Reduce morbidity and mortality	• Increase in staff budget to support clinical audit • Additional nursing time	Clinical audit against key markers, e.g. aspirin, cholesterol, smoking, exercise	• Clinical staff to attend workshop • Reviewing evidence for what is effective in secondary prevention of CHD	High priority Year 1	Review progress at 6/12 month intervals using • audit reviewing workload, • results of audit, workload, • patient satisfaction surveys

OBJECTIVES OF THE PRACTICE

Why was this chosen?	What are we going to do?	How will this benefit our patients?	Do we require any additional resources?	How will we know that we have been successful?	Any need for further training?	Priority	Outcome (clinical audit against key markers)

PART 3
Personal Development

Framework for personal development plans

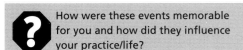

- • Reflect on your practice: past and future.
- • Identify your strengths and weaknesses.
- • Record your agreed plan of action.
- • Review your action plan regularly.
- • Collect evidence of learning in your portfolio.
- • Update it every year.

Does this highlight any gaps and objectives for the future?

How were these events memorable for you and how did they influence your practice/life?

Personal development plans (PDPs) are here to stay, and will play an important part in clinical governance and revalidation. Your PDP is confidential, and should another doctor, such as your GP tutor, see it for revalidation purposes, you may ask him/her to sign a copy of the Confidential Declaration form, see page 163.

A PDP looks at where you wish to be, for example, in the next 5 years: how you will achieve it, what resources you will need and what barriers you will meet.

This section introduces some methods and tools for developing a plan. Many of these will be familiar to trainers and recent GP registrars.

Whichever methods you choose, a simple process is outlined below which may be of help to you in structuring your learning and deciding what could go into your portfolio.

Getting started

We suggest you set aside protected time for this exercise, for which you may be able to gain PGEA accreditation. GPs have busy lives, and it is easy to keep on working without making time to reflect. You can start by reflecting on your past achievements and goals for the future. The guides below can be used to help you move on and develop your PDP.

A past educational profile involves writing down all the educational positions and achievements of your career. A recent curriculum vitae will provide much of this information. You can list your specific educational highlights and achievements. An example of a past educational profile and pro forma can be found on page 126.

The **learning highlights** of the past few years is a simpler method which focuses on specific educational events or workshops which made a real impression on you. You might have learned a new skill, such as joint injections, gained managerial experience, or perhaps learned a new language! An example of how to record your learning highlights and pro forma are on pages 128–9.

A **self-audit** looks at your current situation and where you would like to go. A mentor or partner can augment this process considerably. It includes a personal **SCOT analysis**, (see p. 130) listing your strengths and the challenges, identifying the opportunities for improvement or career progression and noting any threats to such progress.

When you have accomplished the above, you may have identified some major and minor areas of learning and development needs which you may wish to add to your PDP.

PAST EDUCATIONAL PROFILE

Positions	Achievements
Associate GP tutor	Organizing educational events Member of GP Tutor group Liaison with PGEA authorities
Advanced Trainers' Course	Remedial GP training Alternative educational approaches Importance of structure in GP training
Practice prescribing lead	Member of Clinical Governance Group
Member of local Research Ethics Committee	Understanding ethics and research
Group leader at GP Registrars' Day Release Course	Working in small groups

Does this highlight any gaps and objectives for the future?

Gaps	Future objectives
Small group leader training	Further develop my small group skills
Lack of clinical focus	Set up a practice-based journal club
Clinical Governance	Develop practice-based multi-professional learning
IT	Look for appropriate course to attend

PAST EDUCATIONAL PROFILE

Positions	Achievements

Does this highlight any gaps and objectives for the future?

Gaps	Future objectives

LEARNING HIGHLIGHTS

The **learning highlights** of the past few years is a simpler method which focuses on specific educational events or workshops which made a real impression on you. You might have learned a new skill, such as joint injections, travelled or learned a new language or gained managerial experience. How was this event memorable for you and how did it influence your practice?

Key dates	What did you do?	Why?	What did you learn from this?	How have you used this?
February 95	'String of Pearls' Refresher Course	To collect PGEA points	Several disparate pieces of mainly clinical knowledge and management	Implementation in day to day practice
March 96	Palliative Care Course	Elderly population Prevalence of chronic disease	Skills and attitudes relevant to terminal care	Continues to be used regularly
August 97	Sports Medicine	Large student population	Pathophysiology of injury; management of recovery	More appropriate management and use of secondary care
February 98	Travelled to W. Australia	To view any healthcare system in context of that society's culture	That the British NHS is not the only proper way to deliver healthcare	I have maintained contact with Australian GPs since then
June 98	Undertook a 6-week refresher evening course in conversational French	Wanted to go on holiday in France with my family	Learned enough to be able to get by on holiday and found that I had remembered much of my school French	Apart from enjoying our holiday, I would like to continue studying it in more depth and become sufficiently fluent

LEARNING HIGHLIGHTS

The **learning highlights** of the past few years is a simpler method which focuses on specific educational events or workshops which made a real impression on you. You might have learned a new skill, such as joint injections, travelled or learned a new language or gained managerial experience. How was this event memorable for you and how did it influence your practice?

Key dates	What did you do?	Why?	What did you learn from this?	How have you used this?

The self-audit and personal SCOT analysis

It is worth standing back occasionally and looking at who we are, where we are and where we would like to get to. Some people do this at regular intervals, such as birthdays or the start of the year. This has much to recommend it. Whenever it is done, the results can form the basis for rational objective setting, decision-making, planning and action.

Whatever the reason for undertaking a self-audit and personal SCOT analysis, it will always be necessary to be systematic, thorough and objective. This calls for a methodical framework and, if possible, input from at least one other person: a partner, close colleague, mentor, older child, friend or counsellor.

It is always best to work on paper. Some people find a large format, such as flipchart or white board particularly helpful, especially if working with another person. Brainstorm each heading, listing as many possibilities as you can. Look back, refining and editing what you have written, and produce a final, polished listing you can keep and use.

The following checklists may help in the process, although the questions are not by any means exhaustive.

Ask yourself:

What qualifications do I have?

What special knowledge and experience do I have?

What support do I have from family and friends?

In so far as I have succeeded, what has helped me to do so?

What are the sources of my motivation and drive?

Have I any strong, specific interests, at work or outside?

Strengths and challenges are things which exist for you now. Opportunities and threats are possibilities which may come along in the future, but which need to be thought about now. You will need to maximize your strengths and opportunities and minimize your challenges and threats.

?
• Did this highlight any areas that should be added to your PDP?

My strengths (relate to achievements over the year)	**My challenges** (highlight any difficulties or obstacles which have been experienced)

My opportunities (List the factors which will influence your success, i.e. ideas for the future)	**My threats** (Obstacles to development)

Sticky moments
Identifying educational and professional development needs

This is a system that operates by identifying when a problem arising during a consultation is not met because of inadequate skills or knowledge of the doctor. From this can be deduced what the doctor needs to learn so that next time he/she will be better equipped to deal with the problem.

The consultation is the pivotal transaction in general practice and it is during the consultation that one should start to identify learning needs by exploring whether a patient's need has been met. It is important to separate a patient's wants from a patient's needs (they may want a pill for their headache but need to come to terms with an unhappy marriage). It is easy to find out what a doctor wants to learn but much more of a challenge to identify their needs.

How is it done?

After each consultation ask yourself 'Was I equipped to meet the patient's needs?' To answer this question you must home in on the crux of the consultation and ask yourself whether you had the skills and knowledge to deal with it appropriately. You will soon find your first 'sticky moment'. At this point you must decide which category you are dealing with.

Is it?

Clinical knowledge	**CK**
Non-clinical knowledge	**NCK**
Skill	**S**
Attitude	**A**
Practice organization	**PO**

Recording the 'sticky moment' and identifying educational and professional development needs

It is vital that the whole educational process is linked to improving patient care and remains relevant to everyday practice. Try and relate your education needs to a particular clinical situation. Record it on the 'Sticky moments' pro forma (see p. 135), which is totally confidential to you. Keep a copy of this pro forma on your desk so that you are able to record a 'sticky moment' as and when it arises. The process is as follows.

- Make a note of the consultation and the patient ID.
- Describe the sticky moment.
- Identify the educational need.
- Define area for improvement, development or change.
- Classify into category (i.e. CK, NKC, S, A or PO).
- Decide how you are going to meet this need, for example you could:
  Ask a colleague
  Look it up in a textbook
  Medline search
  Journal club
  Practice meetings.

- Describe what you have learned and how it may change your clinical behaviour (see also Reflective practice, p. 12).
- Collect the evidence of what you have learned in your portfolio.

In addition to an individual GP's sticky moments, there may be others which apply to the whole practice. (This is an excellent way of identifying significant events, see p. 60.)

Practice sticky moments and subsequent development needs may support an individual GP's needs, conflict with individual GP's needs or even be irrelevant.

Try to provide at least one example of such an educational need in each category.

Supporting needs	Conflicting needs	Irrelevant needs

PDP?
- Do you need to do anything as a result?
- Would you like to add this to your

Select one example of conflicting needs above. How might this apparent tension in 'needs' be constructively resolved (a GP wishing to take an MSc course that does not form part of the practice plans)?

STICKY MOMENTS

Clinical knowledge	CK
Non-clinical knowledge	NCK
Skill	S
Attitude	A
Practice organization	PO

Date	Patient		The sticky moment	Area for improvement, development or change	Class CK/NCK/S/A/PO
	Age	Sex			
	39	M	History of peptic ulcer, requests triple therapy—which one?	Best 'triple therapy'. Test for H. Pylori? Gastroscopy?	CK
	22	M	Urethral discharge? Refer to GU clinic—how?	Referral criteria and opening times for GU clinic	NCK
	63	F	Persistent tennis elbow. How to inject? When?	Elbow injections	S
	32	M	Became impatient with him, anxiety about job/ redundancy	Don't like men being anxious— want him to pull his socks up	A
	78	F	Consultation went badly— patient waiting more than half an hour in waiting room	Appointment system	PO

STICKY MOMENTS

Clinical knowledge	CK
Non-clinical knowledge	NCK
Skill	S
Attitude	A
Practice organization	PO

Date	Patient		The sticky moment	Area for improvement, development or change	Class CK/NCK/S/A/PO
	Age	Sex			

IDENTIFICATION OF EDUCATIONAL NEEDS

What did I identify as an educational need?	How am I going to meet this need?	What have I learned?	Have I collected the evidence of my learning in my portfolio?	Date completed
Triple therapy for peptic ulcers—which is best?	Medline/library search. Recent review article			
GU Unit details not available in surgery	Secretary to obtain from clinic			
Tennis elbow injection technique	Attend joint injection workshop			
Anxious young man/impatient doctor	Recognize problem of attitude to this kind of patient. Discuss with partner/mentor. Communication workshop			
Patient waiting too long in waiting room	Discuss at partners' meeting. Audit waiting times and consultation interviews			

IDENTIFICATION OF EDUCATIONAL NEEDS

What did I identify as an educational need?	How am I going to meet this need?	What have I learned?	Have I collected the evidence of my learning in my portfolio?	Date completed

Blind spots

You may identify other 'needs' by using this simple checklist of blind spots.

1 Personal skills
   - Communication, e.g. effective and appropriate telephone advice
   - Time management
   - Coping with pressure
   - Challenging patients
   - Finance
   - Personal organization
   - Staff management
   - Navigating the NHS.
2 Clinical skills
   - CPR and other basic clinical skills, e.g. fundoscopy
   - Medical knowledge.
3 New developments in primary care
   - Clinical effectiveness
   - IT and NHS Intranet
   - Clinical audit
   - Research and development
   - PCGs and clinical governance.
4 Local and national priorities
   - Coronary heart disease
   - Stroke
   - Accidents
   - Infection control
   - Mental health
   - Sexual health
   - Chronic disease
   - Substance misuse
   - Ethnicity and health
   - Cancer
   - Elderly
   - Carers
   - New technology
   - Health and safety.

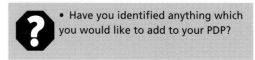

• Have you identified anything which you would like to add to your PDP?

Other methods of identifying needs are discussed in more detail below. You may also identify needs from reading, journal clubs, or internet browsing.

Phased evaluation plan (PEP)

The Royal College of General Practitioners developed 'PEP', a set of educational self-assessment programs for general practice in 1987, principally as a formative assessment tool for GP registrars. It was then made available to any GP who wished to make use of it, with PGEA accreditation available. PEP has proved to be popular and effective as a teaching instrument since its inception with both GPs and those training for general practice. It is widely used by course organizers and trainers both in the UK and abroad and in the Armed Forces. Since that time, there have been many changes in the methods of assessment within the program.

A PEP CD was designed to provide a diagnostic self-assessment tool to establish core knowledge, demonstrate strength and identify areas of deficiency. This can be used to plan further teaching and individual learning.

• Would you like to add this to your PDP?

It can be used on a PC with a CD-rom drive at home or in the surgery and results are confidential.

The PEP CD contains a general practice generic program and 13 speciality programs covering the areas of:

Therapeutics and prescribing	**Emergency medicine**
Asthma	**Family planning**
Practice management	**Geriatric medicine**
General medicine	**Psychiatry**
Dermatology	**Paediatrics**
Obstetrics and gynaecology	**ENT**
Ophthalmology	

To order a CD, contact:
The PEP Office
RCGP
12 Queen Street
Edinburgh
EH2 1JE
Tel: 0131 247 3683/5
Fax: 0131 247 3681

Communication skills

A medical degree is no substitute for clairvoyance.
(George Bernard Shaw)

If you want a guarantee, buy a toaster.
(A rude doctor)

Communication is the final common pathway of everything we do and as society changes, so does our consultation behaviour. In 1871, the American physician Oliver Wendell Holmes told his students 'Your patient has no more right to all the truth you know than he has to all the medicine in your saddlebags ... He should get only so much as is good for him.' As recently as 1993, 60% of European gastroenterologists would not routinely tell a patient he or she had cancer (Thomsen *et al.* 1993), but as we enter a new Millennium, about the only patients protected from their diagnosis are those with dementia (Vassilas & Donaldson 1998). However, in these days of audit and evidence-based medicine, the goalposts are shifting again. Assertive patients want to know not just 'What have I got, doctor?' but 'Will it work, doctor?' and even 'Are you any good at it, doctor?'

The law too is changing as the UK merges with Europe. Out will go the Bolam principle, whereby patients are told what a reasonable doctor considers is right. Instead, patients will have a right to know 'what a reasonable patient would want to know', and who would not want to know if the surgeon you are referring them to is a specialist, with figures to prove it, or a 'once-a-year bodger'? With the advent of clinical audit, it may well be that PCGs will be held responsible, having failed in their duty of care, if the services they purchase turn out to be sub-standard. There are difficult times ahead.

So, how can you keep your communication skills up to scratch? The key unit of accountability for GPs is the primary-care team, and you have to make space for honest, open discussion. Most of the communication problems encountered are not because of difficult patients, but rather difficulties between partners. As a team, you are collectively responsible for the competence of every member, and the days when you could bury or ignore worries about a colleague have gone. Poor communication in a previously happy doctor is often the first sign of stress, depression or addiction. Act before it reaches crisis point.

Assessing the quality of secondary services can be a challenge, but a good unit will already be auditing its work and happy to let you see the results. Perhaps you should discuss these results with your patients before making a referral? Out of necessity, but with some irony, the paediatric cardiac surgery unit at Bristol Children's Hospital has been first to publish its results on the Web on a named surgeon basis (http://www.ubht.org.uk). Communicating such information direct to patients is fraught with difficulty but there is no going back now. Blind trust is being overtaken by informed scepticism.

As for doctor–patient communication, there are several options, each of which requires a fair amount of bravery. In an ideal world, we should scrutinize each other's consulting with the same rigour we scrutinize our prescribing but many of us feel threatened by being directly observed at work. Training practices may have the technology to allow staff (not just the GPs) to video their consultations (with consent) but the key to successful analysis requires constructive feedback, a skill which a few of us are not able to manage intuitively.

However, within your PCG, there are sure to be experienced teachers who could lend their expertise, and your local course organizer, GP tutor or university may offer the resource of simulated patients. These are usually professional actors who are trained not just to assimilate realistically a wide range of patient roles but to give constructive and insightful feedback. They can often be hired out (e.g. for an away day in a congenial setting) and used to reinvent scenarios tailored to individual members of staff. Reflect on what areas you find most difficult, write the scenario and then do it until you feel competent. If it is done well, it can be about the best training there is.

But what about a model of analysis? All of us like the safety blanket of structure, although rarely need to resort to the harness of Pendelton's rules. Brilliant communicators are often 'unconsciously competent' but to reflect on what we are doing and share skills with others we need to be able to articulate what went on. Perhaps the following model may help.

1 Agenda (what were you trying to achieve?).
2 Outcome (what did you think you achieved?).
3 Process (Which skills and tactics worked? Which didn't? Why not? What else might you have done?).
4 Issues (implications for you as a doctor, the team, how you cope with the job, etc.).

A final thought: observation of hundreds of students and doctors communicating over the last 7 years has shown that the really good ones nearly always have two things in common: a life outside medicine and an ability to draw a clear distinction between work and leisure. Workaholism may be the respectable addiction, but it is as damaging as any other, so remember,

- Do you need to take time out to brush up on your consultation skills?
- If so, why don't you add it to your PDP?

no one ever said on their deathbed that they wished they had spent more time at the office.

Medical ethics

Why is study of medical ethics important?

Being a good GP is an odd compound of broad knowledge, multiple skills, deep stickability and a touch of showbiz: but even just to get by we need some understanding of how to make moral judgements. Most dramatically, we need this when there are *conflicts*: a patient makes a difficult demand, partners fall out, or the PCG board faces a choice between two vital services. Most obviously, we need such a skill when faced with *identified dilemmas*: requests for termination of pregnancy or euthanasia, the temptation to lie to a dying patient, an encounter with an uncontrolled epileptic patient who insists on driving. Most commonly, we have *feelings of discomfort,* which alert us to something which is not right in what we are hearing or doing. But in reality almost every choice in healthcare, at any level, has a moral element if we look. A decision made carefully, with options and their logic examined and different players' perspectives taken into account, will be a better decision, while one that is slipshod, imposed, or with arguments and views only partially understood, is bound to be flawed, and may come unstuck. As well as scientific evidence, relevant audit and appropriate clinical skills, we need to be able to detect the moral elements of a problem and weigh them carefully with the other aspects. Call it clinical governance, survival or lifelong learning, it is certainly what good practice is about.

Example

One of your longest serving staff has a new boyfriend who is on the practice list. Late one evening, you leave her to lock up, but return to collect something you have left behind and surprise her reading his notes. Confused and distressed, she discloses that he has been open to her about his previous bisexual lifestyle, but has been evasive when she asked about his previous partners. Someone has just told her that 'someone he was close to had died of AIDS' and she has not been able to sleep or work properly for thinking about it. Unfortunately, she just has her finger on an unguarded and uncomplimentary note made in the records by the new partner.

- What sort of problems trip you up?
- What sort of issues do you have strong views about?
- Would you like to spend some time thinking about these, from different points of view (including those at variance with your own)?
- Would you like to include these in your PDP?

Resuscitation: are you prepared?

Every GP will find they have to manage patients with acute myocardial infarction, and occasionally cardiac arrest. As the latter always occurs in unexpected circumstances, would you be able to cope?

The most common cause of adult sudden cardiac death is ischaemic heart disease, or rhythm abnormalities with no obvious underlying cause. Other important causes are trauma, choking, drug overdose, hypothermia, immersion and anaphylaxis.

Properly managed, survival rates from cardiac arrest, with a good neurological outcome, are of the order of 15–30%.

The key elements for survival

- Immediate call for help (Telephone 999 or 112).
- Immediate bystander basic life support to buy time:
  artificial ventilation through a clear airway;
  external chest compressions.
- Early defibrillation:
  Almost all of the survivors come from those with ventricular fibrillation or pulseless ventricular tachycardia.
  Defibrillation performed early has a very high prospect of success but survival rates fall by 7% for every minute of delay.
  ECG defibrillators are now automated, very simple to use and considerably cheaper than they were.
  In addition to the ambulance service, several police forces, fire services, airlines and elements of the Red Cross and St John Ambulance Association have now been trained and supplied with automated defibrillators.
  There have been many reports of the use of defibrillators by GPs with even higher success rates than the ambulance service.
- Airway management and ventilation with oxygen.
- Essential to prevent hypoxic damage to vital organs if the period of cardiac arrest extends to more than about 4 minutes.
- Drug therapy, with agents such as adrenaline or lidocaine, has little, if any, proven value in improving outcome after cardiac arrest (except for adrenaline in anaphylaxis).

Are you prepared?

There is no more frightening experience for any GP than to be confronted with a patient with a cardiac arrest.

Are you and your staff prepared to respond to such a situation?	❏ Yes/No ❏
When did you last attend a course on resuscitation, or even read about what to do?	❏ Yes/No ❏
Have you arranged for your nurses and your reception staff to attend a course?	❏ Yes/No ❏
Have you acquired posters or leaflets showing what to do in a cardiorespiratory arrest?	❏ Yes/No ❏
Do you know how to operate an ECG defibrillator?	❏ Yes/No ❏
Does your practice have an ECG defibrillator?	❏ Yes/No ❏
Is it not time you acquired one for the emergency doctor?	❏ Yes/No ❏
Do you have oxygen on the premises?	❏ Yes/No ❏
Does the emergency duty doctor carry oxygen?	❏ Yes/No ❏
Do you or your nurses carry adrenaline for anaphylaxis?	❏ Yes/No ❏
Have you arranged for relatives of at risk patients to be trained in basic life support?	❏ Yes/No ❏

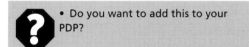

• Do you want to add this to your PDP?

If not, why not?

If you have answered 'No' to most of these questions, ask yourself if your performance would measure up to standards of best practice.

For more information on training opportunities for you and your staff and for information about posters, leaflets and equipment contact the resuscitation officer at your local hospital.

Looking after yourself

There is no doubt that any type of stress or distraction can significantly affect the performance of healthcare professionals to varying degrees. It is a doctor's or nurse's ultimate performance that counts.

It is important to understand the difference between performance and competence. Competence is what a healthcare professional is capable of during an ideal patient consultation on an ideal day. Performance is what the healthcare professional actually does. The difference between one's competence and performance is commonly a function of a distractor, i.e. those things that interfere with ideal function.

Competence = What one is capable of doing
Performance = What one actually does
Performance = Competence – Distractor

Each of us has a variety of coping mechanisms to deal with our individual distractions. These coping mechanisms may vary from time to time. When coping mechanisms are inadequate or overwhelmed the result is distress, impaired performance or both.

What really counts is performance, not competence. The following questionnaires are examples of a tool which may help you identify areas of distraction or competence. Once a person is aware of a problem there may be an opportunity to change. Change often requires a shift in attitude. The ultimate goal is to have healthcare professionals who are happy, healthy and performing well.

Try and identify your priorities both personally and professionally. Take a few minutes to complete the following questionnaire. It is designed to increase awareness of the types of distractors that can interfere with performance and also some of the common coping mechanisms. There is no right or wrong answer or rating scale. Consider each item and become more aware. Perhaps take a risk and share your responses with a trusted colleague. Just discussing some of these issues can make a difference!

> **?** After completing the following questionnaires, have you learned anything about your performance that you may wish to add to your PPDP or PDP?

MANAGING PERFORMANCE DISTRACTORS
SELF-EVALUATION

Reproduced with permission from the College of Physicians and Surgeons of British Colombia and the co-authors, Dr Maureen Piercy and Dr Victor Waymouth.

> **1 Strongly disagree**
> **2 Disagree**
> **3 Neutral**
> **4 Agree**
> **5 Strongly agree**
> **6 Unable to assess**

	1	2	3	4	5	6
1 I enjoy practice as much now as I ever have.	❑	❑	❑	❑	❑	❑
2 I can get locums for my practice for holiday and education time.	❑	❑	❑	❑	❑	❑
3 I am satisfied with my 'on call' schedule.	❑	❑	❑	❑	❑	❑
4 I am satisfied with the total number of hours that I work.	❑	❑	❑	❑	❑	❑
5 I have learned to cope with the 'system' that keeps placing demands on me.	❑	❑	❑	❑	❑	❑
6 I am satisfied with the medical care I provide.	❑	❑	❑	❑	❑	❑
7 I am not fearful of being sued or having a complaint about me.	❑	❑	❑	❑	❑	❑
8 I recognize my limitations and refer patients when I am unsure.	❑	❑	❑	❑	❑	❑
9 I communicate effectively with patients, their families and other health professionals.	❑	❑	❑	❑	❑	❑
10 I show compassion for patients and their families.	❑	❑	❑	❑	❑	❑
11 I produce medical records that are legible and that have enough information to allow a peer to understand my reasoning process for each patient encounter.	❑	❑	❑	❑	❑	❑
12 All those working in my surgery understand and respect patient confidentiality.	❑	❑	❑	❑	❑	❑
13 I am financially secure.	❑	❑	❑	❑	❑	❑
14 I can afford to take off as much time as I need.	❑	❑	❑	❑	❑	❑

	1	2	3	4	5	6
15 I have a plan that will allow me to retire at a selected time.	❏	❏	❏	❏	❏	❏
16 I have no illness that interferes with the quality of my work.	❏	❏	❏	❏	❏	❏
17 I have a GP who is not myself.	❏	❏	❏	❏	❏	❏
18 I exercise at least three times per week.	❏	❏	❏	❏	❏	❏
19 I seldom feel angry or irritable.	❏	❏	❏	❏	❏	❏
20 I manage personal stress effectively.	❏	❏	❏	❏	❏	❏
21 I do not use alcohol or drugs to deal with stress on 'bad days'.	❏	❏	❏	❏	❏	❏
22 I am tolerant of other people and events most of the time.	❏	❏	❏	❏	❏	❏
23 I have a colleague to discuss my problems or concerns with.	❏	❏	❏	❏	❏	❏
24 I have a personal relationship that is supportive.	❏	❏	❏	❏	❏	❏
25 I have interests outside of medicine that I enjoy.	❏	❏	❏	❏	❏	❏
26 I am still learning, growing, gaining new perspectives and not feeling stagnant.	❏	❏	❏	❏	❏	❏
27 I recognize the difference between the things I cannot control or change and those things I can influence.	❏	❏	❏	❏	❏	❏
28 Reflecting on my career, I feel satisfied that my contribution has 'made a difference' and that there is purpose and meaning to my life.	❏	❏	❏	❏	❏	❏
29 I set aside time on a regular basis to grow emotionally and spiritually.	❏	❏	❏	❏	❏	❏
30 I am content with my life at this time.	❏	❏	❏	❏	❏	❏

THE WORK OF GENERAL PRACTICE
QUESTIONNAIRE

Key	
1	**I feel very confident about this.**
2	**I feel quite confident about this.**
3	**I need to learn a bit about this.**
4	**I need to learn a lot about this.**

Questionnaire to measure your confidence in dealing with the following conditions

	1	2	3	4
Infectious diseases				
Childhood infections	❑	❑	❑	❑
Influenza	❑	❑	❑	❑
Gastroenteritis	❑	❑	❑	❑
Pyrexia of unknown origin	❑	❑	❑	❑
Glandular fever	❑	❑	❑	❑
Hepatitis A	❑	❑	❑	❑
Hepatitis B	❑	❑	❑	❑
HIV	❑	❑	❑	❑
Tropical disease	❑	❑	❑	❑
Travel jabs	❑	❑	❑	❑
Notifiable disease	❑	❑	❑	❑
'Free from Infection' certificate	❑	❑	❑	❑
Evidence-based use of antibiotics	❑	❑	❑	❑
Ear, nose & throat				
Facial pain	❑	❑	❑	❑
Catarrhal child	❑	❑	❑	❑
Otitis media	❑	❑	❑	❑
Glue ear	❑	❑	❑	❑
Tonsillitis/Sore throat	❑	❑	❑	❑
Sinusitis	❑	❑	❑	❑
Deafness	❑	❑	❑	❑
Audiology/Hearing aids	❑	❑	❑	❑
Hoarseness	❑	❑	❑	❑
Ménière's disease	❑	❑	❑	❑
Vertigo	❑	❑	❑	❑
Tinnitus	❑	❑	❑	❑
Hay fever	❑	❑	❑	❑
Indications for T&A	❑	❑	❑	❑
Dysphagia	❑	❑	❑	❑
Epistaxis	❑	❑	❑	❑
Eyes				
Conjunctivitis	❑	❑	❑	❑
Painful red eye	❑	❑	❑	❑
Corneal ulcers	❑	❑	❑	❑
Cataract	❑	❑	❑	❑
Squint/orthoptics	❑	❑	❑	❑
Glaucoma	❑	❑	❑	❑
Fundoscopy	❑	❑	❑	❑

	1	2	3	4
Services for partial sight	❑	❑	❑	❑
Sudden loss of vision	❑	❑	❑	❑
Floaters	❑	❑	❑	❑
Chest and breast diseases				
Acute asthma	❑	❑	❑	❑
Chronic asthma	❑	❑	❑	❑
COPD	❑	❑	❑	❑
Occupational lung diseases	❑	❑	❑	❑
TB	❑	❑	❑	❑
Bronchitis/Pneumonia	❑	❑	❑	❑
Ca lung	❑	❑	❑	❑
Cough	❑	❑	❑	❑
Acute breathlessness	❑	❑	❑	❑
Screening for Ca breast	❑	❑	❑	❑
Chest pain (excl. cardiovascular)	❑	❑	❑	❑
Heart and circulation				
Hypertension	❑	❑	❑	❑
Lipids	❑	❑	❑	❑
Heart failure	❑	❑	❑	❑
Acute MI	❑	❑	❑	❑
Angina	❑	❑	❑	❑
CPR	❑	❑	❑	❑
Post-MI rehabilitation	❑	❑	❑	❑
ECGs	❑	❑	❑	❑
Peripheral vascular disease	❑	❑	❑	❑
Varicose veins	❑	❑	❑	❑
Deep vein thrombosis	❑	❑	❑	❑
Collapse	❑	❑	❑	❑
Primary prevention of heart disease	❑	❑	❑	❑
Secondary prevention of heart disease	❑	❑	❑	❑
Gynaecology/genitourinary				
Menopause/HRT	❑	❑	❑	❑
Cervical screening	❑	❑	❑	❑
Breast screening	❑	❑	❑	❑
Post-menopausal bleeding	❑	❑	❑	❑
Vaginal discharge	❑	❑	❑	❑
Dyspareunia	❑	❑	❑	❑
Impotence	❑	❑	❑	❑
Subfertility	❑	❑	❑	❑
Psychosexual problems	❑	❑	❑	❑
RELATE	❑	❑	❑	❑
Cystitis	❑	❑	❑	❑
Nephritis/Pyelitis	❑	❑	❑	❑
Renal colic	❑	❑	❑	❑
Haematuria	❑	❑	❑	❑
Uterine/Ovarian cancer	❑	❑	❑	❑
Bladder/Prostatic cancer	❑	❑	❑	❑
Prostatism/Retention	❑	❑	❑	❑
Incontinent males	❑	❑	❑	❑
Incontinent females	❑	❑	❑	❑

	1	2	3	4
Family planning				
Oral contraception	❑	❑	❑	❑
Other hormonal methods	❑	❑	❑	❑
Caps	❑	❑	❑	❑
IUCD	❑	❑	❑	❑
Sterilization	❑	❑	❑	❑
Other contraceptive methods	❑	❑	❑	❑
Under 16s	❑	❑	❑	❑
Religious/Ethnic differences	❑	❑	❑	❑
Unplanned pregnancy & TOP	❑	❑	❑	❑
Obstetrics				
Antenatal care in practice	❑	❑	❑	❑
Postnatal care in practice	❑	❑	❑	❑
Home deliveries	❑	❑	❑	❑
Administration (forms/benefits/claims)	❑	❑	❑	❑
Paediatrics				
Child health surveillance	❑	❑	❑	❑
Common minor problems	❑	❑	❑	❑
Minor orthopaedic problems	❑	❑	❑	❑
Common acute emergencies	❑	❑	❑	❑
Rare but important emergencies	❑	❑	❑	❑
GP role in rare disease	❑	❑	❑	❑
Behavioural problems (Sources of help)	❑	❑	❑	❑
Children Act (Physical/Sexual abuse)	❑	❑	❑	❑
Child protection/Courts	❑	❑	❑	❑
Adoption/Fostering/Residential homes	❑	❑	❑	❑
The elderly				
Over-75 health surveillance	❑	❑	❑	❑
Falls in the elderly	❑	❑	❑	❑
Dementia	❑	❑	❑	❑
Elderly in own homes	❑	❑	❑	❑
Residential/Nursing homes	❑	❑	❑	❑
Home carers	❑	❑	❑	❑
Meals on Wheels	❑	❑	❑	❑
Voluntary services and private sector	❑	❑	❑	❑
Cancer				
Early recognition/Screening	❑	❑	❑	❑
Symptom relief/Palliative care	❑	❑	❑	❑
GP knowledge of hospital care	❑	❑	❑	❑
Role of hospice/Macmillan nurse	❑	❑	❑	❑
Communication with patients/relatives	❑	❑	❑	❑
Abdomen				
Recurrent upper abdominal pain	❑	❑	❑	❑
Recurrent lower abdominal pain	❑	❑	❑	❑
Acute abdominal pain	❑	❑	❑	❑
Diarrhoea	❑	❑	❑	❑
Indication for investigation	❑	❑	❑	❑
Rectal bleeding	❑	❑	❑	❑
Weight loss	❑	❑	❑	❑
Central nervous system				
Epilepsy	❑	❑	❑	❑

	1	2	3	4
Hysterical fits	❏	❏	❏	❏
Headache	❏	❏	❏	❏
Migraine	❏	❏	❏	❏
Parkinson's disease	❏	❏	❏	❏
CVA/TIA	❏	❏	❏	❏
Stroke rehabilitation	❏	❏	❏	❏
MS	❏	❏	❏	❏
Brain tumours	❏	❏	❏	❏
·TATT	❏	❏	❏	❏

Endocrine disease

	1	2	3	4
Managing diabetes	❏	❏	❏	❏
Complication of diabetes	❏	❏	❏	❏
GP diabetic clinics	❏	❏	❏	❏
Hypothyroidism	❏	❏	❏	❏
Hyperthyroidism	❏	❏	❏	❏
Hyperprolactinaemia	❏	❏	❏	❏
Delayed puberty	❏	❏	❏	❏

Musculoskeletal

	1	2	3	4
Rheumatoid	❏	❏	❏	❏
Osteoarthritis	❏	❏	❏	❏
Gout	❏	❏	❏	❏
Osteoporosis	❏	❏	❏	❏
Back pain	❏	❏	❏	❏
Neck/Shoulder pain	❏	❏	❏	❏
Physiotherapy	❏	❏	❏	❏
Local injections	❏	❏	❏	❏
Tendon inflammation	❏	❏	❏	❏
Complementary medicine	❏	❏	❏	❏
ME/Fibromyalgia	❏	❏	❏	❏
Joint injections	❏	❏	❏	❏
Peri-articular injection	❏	❏	❏	❏

Diseases of the mind

	1	2	3	4
Anxiety	❏	❏	❏	❏
Depression	❏	❏	❏	❏
Insomnia	❏	❏	❏	❏
Atypical presentations of depression	❏	❏	❏	❏
Abuse of prescribed drugs	❏	❏	❏	❏
Abuse of illicit drugs	❏	❏	❏	❏
Alcohol abuse	❏	❏	❏	❏
Smoking	❏	❏	❏	❏
Eating disorders	❏	❏	❏	❏
Managing the disturbed patient	❏	❏	❏	❏
Counselling	❏	❏	❏	❏
Family therapy	❏	❏	❏	❏
Mental health team	❏	❏	❏	❏
Care in the community	❏	❏	❏	❏

Skin disease

	1	2	3	4
Acne	❏	❏	❏	❏
Eczema	❏	❏	❏	❏
Psoriasis	❏	❏	❏	❏
Warts	❏	❏	❏	❏

	1	2	3	4
Skin disease (continued)				
Infestations	❏	❏	❏	❏
Fungal infections	❏	❏	❏	❏
Leg ulcers	❏	❏	❏	❏
Skin cancer	❏	❏	❏	❏
Urticaria/Angioedema	❏	❏	❏	❏
Pruritus	❏	❏	❏	❏
Rosacea	❏	❏	❏	❏
Emollients	❏	❏	❏	❏
Drug rashes	❏	❏	❏	❏
In-growing toenails	❏	❏	❏	❏
Sebaceous cysts	❏	❏	❏	❏
Skin biopsy	❏	❏	❏	❏
Incision of abscess	❏	❏	❏	❏
Treating warts	❏	❏	❏	❏
Minor surgery—Organization & equipment	❏	❏	❏	❏
Minor surgery—Competence & accreditation	❏	❏	❏	❏
Investigation				
X-ray (use and abuse)	❏	❏	❏	❏
Availability (e.g. Ba enema)	❏	❏	❏	❏
Endoscopy	❏	❏	❏	❏
Ultrasound	❏	❏	❏	❏
Therapeutics				
Practice formularies	❏	❏	❏	❏
Doctor's emergency drugs	❏	❏	❏	❏
PACT	❏	❏	❏	❏
Role of pharmacist	❏	❏	❏	❏
Product liability	❏	❏	❏	❏
Monitoring repeat prescribing	❏	❏	❏	❏
Alternatives to drugs	❏	❏	❏	❏
Generic/Branded private	❏	❏	❏	❏
POM/P	❏	❏	❏	❏
General/Black list	❏	❏	❏	❏
ACBS	❏	❏	❏	❏
Cost–benefit analysis	❏	❏	❏	❏
Controlled drug regulations	❏	❏	❏	❏
Prescription charges/Exemptions	❏	❏	❏	❏
Personally administered items	❏	❏	❏	❏
Disability & handicap				
Medical certificates	❏	❏	❏	❏
Disability Resettlement Officer	❏	❏	❏	❏
Maternity benefit	❏	❏	❏	❏
Sickness benefits	❏	❏	❏	❏
Invalidity benefits	❏	❏	❏	❏
Disability benefits	❏	❏	❏	❏
Attendance allowance (+ special rules)	❏	❏	❏	❏
Mobility Allowance/Motability	❏	❏	❏	❏
Disease oriented groups	❏	❏	❏	❏
Self-help groups	❏	❏	❏	❏

	1	2	3	4
Caring for carers	❏	❏	❏	❏
Residential homes for children/young adults	❏	❏	❏	❏
Fitness to drive	❏	❏	❏	❏
Fit to travel by air	❏	❏	❏	❏

Organization of the NHS

	1	2	3	4
NHS Executive	❏	❏	❏	❏
Health authority	❏	❏	❏	❏
Statement of fees and allowances	❏	❏	❏	❏
Purchaser/Provider split	❏	❏	❏	❏
Patient's Charter	❏	❏	❏	❏
Primary-care group	❏	❏	❏	❏
Clinical governance	❏	❏	❏	❏
LMC	❏	❏	❏	❏
GMC	❏	❏	❏	❏
GPC	❏	❏	❏	❏
CHC	❏	❏	❏	❏
CHIMP	❏	❏	❏	❏
NICE	❏	❏	❏	❏
Community (GP) hospitals	❏	❏	❏	❏
Role of practice managers	❏	❏	❏	❏
Role of practice nurses	❏	❏	❏	❏
Role of health visitors	❏	❏	❏	❏
Role of district nurses	❏	❏	❏	❏
Role of community midwives	❏	❏	❏	❏
Nurse triage/NHS Direct	❏	❏	❏	❏
Co-ops/Deputizing services	❏	❏	❏	❏
Contacting doctors (bleeps, etc.)	❏	❏	❏	❏

Practice organization

	1	2	3	4
Accounts and taxation	❏	❏	❏	❏
Partnership agreement	❏	❏	❏	❏
Appointments systems	❏	❏	❏	❏
Types of patient records	❏	❏	❏	❏
Registers of age/sex or morbidity	❏	❏	❏	❏
Recall systems	❏	❏	❏	❏
Audit	❏	❏	❏	❏
Use of computers	❏	❏	❏	❏
Continuing Education PGEA	❏	❏	❏	❏
Types of practice	❏	❏	❏	❏
Employing staff, contracts, appraisal	❏	❏	❏	❏
Health and Safety at Work	❏	❏	❏	❏
NHS funding for surgery premises	❏	❏	❏	❏
Managing time	❏	❏	❏	❏
Managing change	❏	❏	❏	❏
Managing stress	❏	❏	❏	❏
Complaints	❏	❏	❏	❏
Non-principals	❏	❏	❏	❏
Use of Internet	❏	❏	❏	❏

Prevention, screening, patient education

	1	2	3	4
Criteria for a screening test	❏	❏	❏	❏
Opportunistic screening/Case finding	❏	❏	❏	❏

	1	2	3	4
Prevention, screening, patient education (continued)				
Our Healthier Nation	❑	❑	❑	❑
Targets	❑	❑	❑	❑
Practice leaflet	❑	❑	❑	❑
Newsletter	❑	❑	❑	❑
Medical ethics				
Confidentiality (Relatives/Insurers/ Police, etc.)	❑	❑	❑	❑
Minors (contraception)	❑	❑	❑	❑
Consent to treatment	❑	❑	❑	❑
Euthanasia	❑	❑	❑	❑
Rationing care	❑	❑	❑	❑
TOP	❑	❑	❑	❑
Ethics committee and research	❑	❑	❑	❑
Chaperones	❑	❑	❑	❑
Dispensing by GPs	❑	❑	❑	❑

Meeting educational and development needs

Now that you will have identified your educational and development needs, you may wish to consider ways of meeting these needs. Remember that everyone learns in different ways. We can assimilate information *didactically*, e.g. in lectures, or *experientially* in our work.

Formal and informal methods

Many methods can be valuable, such as:

- Lectures
- Workshops
- Small-group work
  Young principals
  Peer support groups
- Practice meetings
- Clinical assistantships/Individual attachments
- Clinical audits
- Research
- Journal club
- Medline/Internet searches
- Using e-mail
- Distance learning courses
- Individual reading
- Appraisal
- Working in another practice
- Working with other professionals
- Diploma or Masters courses.

This list is by no means exhaustive and some other methods are discussed in more detail on the following pages.

Mentoring

Mentoring is defined as:

> The process whereby an experienced, highly regarded, empathic person (the mentor) guides another individual (the mentee) in the development and re-examination of their own ideas, learning, and personal and professional development. The mentor, who often but not necessarily works in the same organization or field as the mentee, achieves this by listening and talking in confidence to the mentee.

Mentoring can form a valuable part of a framework of support for GPs but should be entirely voluntary and not imposed, with confidentiality an essential part of the process. Both mentors and mentees should fully understand the purpose and limits of the mentoring relationship, and those volunteering to become mentors should be given appropriate assistance to develop their skills. Associate Directors and GP tutors may be contacted for advice.

Different kinds of support are likely to be needed at different points in someone's career. Extra support may well be necessary for newly appointed GPs but can also be valuable for other members of the PHCT.

A suitable time and place is important, and thought should be given to building appropriate amounts of time into people's work programmes. The length and frequency of mentoring meetings is likely to depend on individual needs and preferences.

Mentoring must be separate from the external monitoring and assessment of performance, promotion and remuneration.

Self-directed learning groups

Many GPs may be familiar with this style of working in preparation for the MRCGP examination.

Essentially, a small group (ideally four or five) of like-minded GPs may wish to meet on a regular basis to share some of the workload of meeting their educational needs. This may also be particularly relevant to non-principals who may not regularly have the opportunity to ruminate over clinical situations in a practice setting.

The group could decide which needs may be met. Examples could be:
* researching evidence-based topics;
* therapeutics;
* journal review; and
* case discussion, e.g. clinical, ethical, etc.

It may be appropriate for each group member in turn to prepare material in advance.

Non-principals

Non-principals are an important and growing part of the GP workforce, comprising:
* assistants;
* locums;
* retainer scheme doctors; and
* GP registrars.

Wherever possible, non-principals should be invited to participate and contribute to team activities, such as significant-event auditing, team away days and PPDPs. Although non-principals may lose remuneration through attending these, they can gain much insight into primary care and enhance their personal portfolios and lifelong learning; the team will gain by the fresh insights non-principals can bring.

Non-principals should build on their registrar workbook or portfolio to develop the concept of lifelong learning, use the PDP section of this book, and attend as many team events as they can, recording these using reflective practice principles. This living, ongoing record of lifelong learning will stand them in good stead with the eventual introduction of revalidation.

Portfolio careers

Portfolio careers are a concept familiar to many GPs. A portfolio career GP frequently spends time outside the practice in activities that use a broad range of skills in different environments. Examples are occupational health work, course organization, medical politics, school health clinics and sports medicine.

A portfolio changes over time as new interests are picked up and others dropped to make space. Work patterns also change to fit in with family and other activities. Indeed portfolio careers allow flexibility in working patterns and interests and depend on an ability to reflect on skills and strengths rather than roles. Variation in workplaces and changes in tasks maintain interest and enthusiasm.

There are downsides, as a portfolio career usually means less security. Working with different people can be fun, but it means working on more than one set of relationships.

Continuing professional development and portfolio careers

The standard format of appraisal and job planning may not fit comfortably with a portfolio career. However, a mentor who is willing to spend time with you can be extremely effective. Considering your portfolio at regular intervals gives the opportunity to reflect on the new skills gained and how they might be used in other areas. It also gives an opportunity to consider career moves and how additions to a career portfolio will strengthen your c.v. It is important to be honest about aspirations, and realistic about flexibility. Building up skills that could lead in more than one direction prevents focus into one career path. The same principles apply as to any other professional development.

- What do I want to achieve in the next year?
- How will it fit in with my current role in the NHS?
- What additional knowledge and skills do I want to learn?
- How will I measure success?

The difference may be that some of the new skills may be learned through working in a new area or by expanding an existing area. Two additional questions might be asked.

- Are there new opportunities coming up that I might apply for?
- What could I stop doing to make the time for the new opportunity?

General practice lends itself to portfolio careers; however, it is easy to allow them to develop without too much planning. This can be the cause of disagreements and disgruntlement in the practice and if you are contemplating building your own portfolio, consider the options available to you and how you might build towards an overall goal.

Keeping up to date

This is not easy. Reading the entire contents of this book would take you quite a time. We have to keep up to date, our peers and our patients expect us to and surely it is a matter of professional pride to be abreast of medical developments. There is no easy answer to the problem of how to do it. We need to find the time to browse the journals, but fitting it into the busy work schedule is not easy. Only you can arrange your timetable for this.

- There are innumerable journals available. The classic heavyweights such as the *British Medical Journal* and the *British Journal of General Practice* are obvious choices for the reader. However, there are a number of regular review journals such as *Update*, *Medical Monitors* and many others which give information on current clinical practice or review articles. There are so many to choose from that personal preference is what matters.

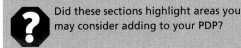
Did these sections highlight areas you may consider adding to your PDP?

- Gather a collection of articles that are of interest and build them into a personal reference library.
- Run a journal club on a regular basis in-house or with other practitioner groups. This generates interest and feedback can be useful.
- Get reports from partners who have perhaps attended a course or conference. Often we can get a distillation of new ideas and procedures, which can be very useful for all.
- Use the Internet. More and more websites are available which include access to specified journals. Using your local health authority website can get you enrolled on the Cochrane Database (see p. 175). This database is very extensive and offers information based on evidence.
- Patients will often ask about new treatments that they have seen reported in the newspapers, on TV or have read about on the Internet. This offers stimulus to find out more about these new concepts. Useful websites can be found on page 175.
- In practice, we are often faced with problems for which there is no immediate answer. These are collectively known as sticky moments as described on page 132. Where there are obvious blanks, be they large or small, make a note of them for answering later.
- Your local PGMC library and others offer help with searches and other references.
- Representatives often have a lot of information on specific subjects and handouts can be quite informative.
- We learn and keep ahead in different ways. There is no hard and fast rule about how to do this, only to recognize the need to manage your own learning in the best way to suit you.

- How are you planning to keep up to date?
- How much time are you prepared to commit?
- How will you collect the evidence of your reading?
- Are you going to include this in your PDP?

The personal development plan

> The list on the following pages is a template of all the relevant sections in this manual. Use it to bring forward anything, which you have identified as being suitable to add to your PDP on page 160.

You may now wish to write your personal development plan (PDP) by considering all the sections in this manual, which may have helped you to identify your educational and development needs. These will form an important link to the practice professional development plan (PPDP).

PERSONAL DEVELOPMENT PLAN

	What is the key thing I have identified?	What is my goal?	How am I going to tackle this	Target date	What will hinder me	Action needed
Past educational profile						
Learning highlights of the past few years						
Self-audit and personal SCOT analysis						
Sticky moments						
Blind spots						
Phased evaluation plan (PEP)						
Communication skills						
Medical ethics						
Resuscitation: are you prepared?						
Looking after yourself						
Mentoring						
Self-directed learning groups						
Non-principals						
Portfolio career						
Keeping up to date						

Did any areas from the PPDP highlight any personal educational and development needs?						
	What is the key thing I have identified?	What is my goal?	How am I going to tackle this?	Target date	What will hinder me?	Action needed
Significant-event auditing						
Using evidence in the management of common diseases						
Audit						
Using complaints to improve practice						
You and your practice						
Referral data						
PACT—prescribing						
Performance indicators in primary care						
Research and development						
Staff appraisals						
Partner review system						

Appendix 1: Confidentiality declaration

I give permission for my Personal Development Plan to be seen for assessment and revalidation purposes by

Dr ....
who will be responsible for the security and confidentiality of my Personal Development Plan, whilst in his/her care.

This permission has been granted on the strict understanding that he/she will not copy any part of my Personal Development Plan, nor divulge any information contained therein, to another party.

Signed: ....
(Submitting Doctor)

Name

Address

Signed: ....
(Assessing Doctor)

Name

Address

Appendix 2: Useful telephone numbers and addresses

Association of British Pharmaceutical Industry (ABPI)	12 Whitehall London SW1A 2DY Tel: 0171 930 3477
Association of Independent Specialist Medical Accountants	48 St Leonard's Road Bexhill-on-Sea Sussex TN40 1JB Tel: 01424 730345
Association of Managers in General Practice (AMGP)	Suite 308 The Foundry 156 Blackfriars Road London SE1 8EN Tel/Fax: 0171 721 7090
Audit Commission	1 Vincent Square London SW1P 2PN Tel: 0171 828 1212 Fax: 0171 976 6187 Website: http://www.auditcommission.gov.uk
British Heart Foundation	14 Fitzhardinge Street London W1H 4DH Tel: 0171 935 0185 Fax: 0171 486 5820 Website: http://www.bhf.org.uk
British Medical Association	BMA House Tavistock House London WC1H 9JP Tel: 0171 387 4499 Fax: 0171 383 6406

British Nursing Association	87A Crane Street Salisbury Wiltshire SP1 2PU Tel: 01722 330551 Fax: 01722 411630
Centre for Evidence Based Medicine	Radcliffe Hospital NHS Trust Headley Way Headington Oxford OX3 9DU Tel: 01865 741166 Fax: 01865 741408
College of Health	St Margarets House 21 Old Ford Road London E2 9PL Tel: 0181 983 1225 Fax: 0181 983 1553 e-mail: info@TCOH.demon.co.uk
Data Protection Register	Springfield House Water Lane Wilmslow Cheshire SK9 5AX Tel: (enquiries) 01625 535777 Tel: (administration) 01625 535711
Department of Health	PO Box 777 London SE1 6XH Tel: 0800 555777 Fax: 01623 724524 Website: http://www.doh.gov.uk
DHSS	Alexander Fleming House Elephant & Castle London SE1 6BH Tel: 0171 820 5800
Faculty of Family Planning	19 Cornwall Terrace London NW1 4QP Tel: 0171 935 7514 Fax: 0171 935 8613 e-mail: mail@ffprhc.org.uk

Family Health Service Appeals
Authority

30 Victoria Avenue
Harrogate
North Yorkshire
HG1 5PR
Tel: 01423 530280
Fax: 01423 522034

Family Planning Association

2–12 Pentonville Road
London
N1 9SP
Tel: 0171 837 5432
Fax: 020 7837 3042
E-mail: margeretmcg@fpa.org.uk
Website: http://www.fpa.org.uk

General Medical Council

178 Great Portland Street
London
W1N 6JE
Tel: 0171 580 7642
Fax: 0171 915 3641
e-mail: gmc@gmc-uk.org
Website: http://www.gmc-uk.org

General Practice Finance
Corporation

Tavistock House (North)
Tavistock Square
London
WC1H 9JL
Tel: 0171 387 5274

General Practice Link Office

Croydon Post Graduate Medical
Centre
Mayday University Hospital
London Road
Croydon
Surrey
CR7 7YE
Tel: 0181 401 3990
Fax: 0181 401 3989

GMPAC

Glasgow Local Medical Committee
40 New City Road
Glasgow
G4 9JT
Tel: 0141 332 8081
Fax: 0141 332 6798
e-mail: bw@glasgow-lmc.co.uk

Health Education Authority

Hamilton House
London
WC1H 9TX
Tel: 0171 383 3833

Health & Safety Executive (HSE) Library & Information Services	Baynards House 1 Chepstow Place Wesbourne Grove London W2 4TF Tel: 0171 221 0870
Health Visitors Association	36 Eccleston Square London SW1V 1PF Tel: 0171 834 9523
Her Majesty's Stationery Office (HMSO)	49 High Holborn London WC1V 6HB Tel: 0171 873 0011
Institute of Health Service Management	7–10 Chandos Street London W1M 9DE Tel: 0171 460 7654 Fax: 0171 460 7655 e-mail: mailbox@ihsm.co.uk Website: http://www.ihsm.co.uk
Institute of Health Service Managers	39 Charlton Street London NW1 1JD Tel: 0171 388 2626 Fax: 0171 388 2386
Joint Committee for Continuing Education of Practice Staff	Tavistock House (North) Tavistock Square London WC1N 9LN Tel: 0171 387 6005
Joint Committee for Postgraduate Training for General Practice	14 Princes Gate Hyde Park London SW7 1PU Tel: 0171 581 3232 Fax: 0171 225 3047 e-mail: info@rcgp.org.uk Website: http://www.rcgp.org.uk

King's Fund

11–13 Cavendish Square
London
W1M 0AN
Tel: 0171 307 2400
Fax: 0171 307 2801
e-mail: library@kingsfund.org.uk
Website:
http://www.kingsfund.org.uk

King's Fund Centre

126 Albert Street
London
NW1 7NF
Tel: 0171 267 6111

Macmillan Cancer Relief

Anchor House
15-19 Britten Street
London
SW3 3TZ
Tel: 0171 351 7811
Fax: 0171 376 8098
Website:
http://www.macmillan.org.uk

Marie Curie Training

17 Grosvenor Crescent
London
SW1 7XZ
Tel: 0171 201 2312
Fax: 0171 235 2243

Medical Defence Union

3 Devonshire Place
London
W1N 2EA
Tel: 0171 486 6181
Advisory services:
Tel: 0800 716646
Fax: 0171 935 5503

Medical Insurance Agency

BMA House
Tavistock Square
London
WC1H 9J9
Tel: 0171 388 1301

Medical Practices Committee

1st Floor, Eileen House
80–94 Newington Causeway
London
SE1 6EF
Tel: 0171 972 2930
Fax: 0171 972 2985
Website: http://www.open.gov.uk/
doh/mpc/mpch.htm

Medical Protection Society Ltd	50 Hallam Street London W1N 6DE Tel: 0171 636 0690 Fax: 0171 637 0541
Medical Research Council	20 Park Crescent London W1N 4AL Tel: 0171 636 5422 Fax: 0171 436 6179 Website: http://www.mrc.ac.uk
Medicines Resource Centre (MeRec)	Mersey RHA Hamilton House 24 Pall Mall Liverpool L3 6AL Tel: 0151 236 4620 ext: 2096
Mental Health Act Commission	Maid Marion House 56 Hounds Gate Nottingham NG1 6BG Tel: 0115 943 7100 Fax: 0115 943 7101 e-mail: chief.executive@ms.mhac.trent.nhs.uk
MIND	Kathleen Aitken 1 Regent Circus Swindon Wiltshire Tel: 01793 432031 Fax: 01793 436889
National Advice Centre for Postgraduate Medical Education	The Health Department Bridgewater House 58 Whitworth Street Manchester M1 6BB Tel: 0161 957 7218 Fax: 0161 957 7029 Website: http://www.britishcouncil.org

National Association of GP Tutors	17 Spring Lane Radcliffe Manchester M26 2TQ Fax: 0161 724 6927 e-mail nagpt@btinternet.com Website http://www.nagpt.org.uk
National Association of Non-Principals	PO Box 188 West Sussex PO19 2ZA Fax: 01243 536428 e-mail info@nanp.org.uk Website http://www.nanp.org.uk
National Association of Patient Participation	Mr Joe Corkill 9 Lymington Road Wallasey Merseyside Tel/Fax: 0151 630 5786
National Asthma & Respiratory Training Centre	Athenaeum 10 Church Street Warwick CV34 4AB Tel: 01926 493313 Fax: 01926 493224 e-mail: enquires@nartc.org.uk Website: http://www.nartc.org.uk
National Asthma Campaign	Provident House Provident Place London N1 0NT Tel: 0171 226 2260 Fax: 0171 704 0740 Website: http://www.asthma.org.co.uk
NHS Executive	Department of Health Quarry House Quarry Hill Leeds LS2 7UE Tel: 0113 254 5610

National Counselling Service for Sick Doctors	First Assist Wheatfield Way Hinckley Leicestershire LE10 1YG Tel: 08702 410535 Fax: 01455 254027
National Institute for Clinical Excellence	90 Long Acre Covent Garden London WCTE 9RF Tel: 0171 383 6451 Fax: 0171 849 3127 e-mail: nice@nice.nhs.uk
National Primary Care Research and Development Centre	5th Floor, Williamson Building University of Manchester Oxford Road Manchester M13 9PL Tel: 0161 275 7601 Fax: 0161 275 7600 Website: http://www.npcrdc.man.ac.uk
Open University	Chilton House 70 Manchester Road Chilton-Come-Hardy Manchester M21 9UN Tel: 0161 861 9823 Fax: 0161 956 6811 Website: http://www.open.ac.uk
Prescription Pricing Authority	Bridge House 152 Pilgrim Street Newcastle upon Tyne NE1 6SN Tel: 0191 232 5371 Fax: 0191 232 2480 *Information Services*: Scottish Life House Archbold Terrace Jesmond Newcastle upon Tyne NE2 1DB Tel: 0191 203 5000 Fax: 0191 203 5001 Website: http://www.pp.nhs.uk

Royal College of General Practitioners	14 Princes Gate Hyde Park London SW7 1PU Tel: 0171 581 3232 Fax: 0171 225 2389 Website: http://www.rcgp.org.uk
Royal College of Nursing	194 Euston Road London NW1 2DA Tel: 0171 409 3333 Fax: 0171 647 3435 Website: http://www.rcn.org.uk
Sainsbury Centre for Mental Health	1340150138 Borough High Street London SE1 1LB Tel: 0171 403 8790 Fax: 0171 403 9482 Website: http://www.sainsburycentre.org.uk
School for Social Entrepreneurs	18 Victoria Park Square Bethnal Green London E2 9PF Tel: 0181 980 6263 Fax: 0181 983 4655 e-mail: info@sse.org.uk Website: http://www.sse.org.uk
SCOPE	6 Market Road London N7 9PW Tel: 0171 619 7100 Fax: 0171 619 7399
SENSE	The National Deaf/Blind & Rubella Association 11–13 Clifton Terrace Finsbury Park London N4 3SR Tel: 0171 272 7774 Fax: 0171 272 6012 Website: http://www.sense.org.uk

The Patients Association

18 Victoria Park Square
Bethnal Green
London
E2 9PF
Tel: 0181 423 8999

UKCC

23 Portland Place
London
W1N 4JT
Tel: 0171 637 7181
Fax: 0171 436 2924
Website: http://www.ukcc.org.uk

LOCAL NAMES AND TELEPHONE NUMBERS FOR PERSONAL COMPLETION

	Contact Person	Telephone Number	E-mail
ACAS			
Associate Director GP Education			
BMA Regional Office			
Clinical Governance Lead			
Director of GP Education			
GP Tutor			
Health Authority			
LMC			
Local Hospital			
Chief Executive Local Primary Care Group			
Medical Insurance Agency Regional Office			
NHS Direct			
NHSE Regional Office			
Postgraduate Centre Administrator			
RCGP Faculty			
University Department of General Practice			
Vocational Training Course and Scheme Organizer			
Walk-in Centre			

Appendix 3: Useful websites

Medline	http://ovid.bma.org.uk
Bandolier	http://www.jr2.ox.ac.uk/Bandolier
Biomednet search page	http://www.biomednet.com
British Medical Journal	http://www.bmj.com
CASP	http://www.phru.org/casp/review.html
Centre for EBM	http://cebm.jr2.ox.ac.uk/
Cochrane	http://www.update-software.com/ccweb/default.html
Doctor's Desk	http://drsdesk.sghms.ac.uk
Education for General Practice	http://www.educationgp.com
Evidence Based Health	http://www.mailbase.ac.uk/lists/evidence-based-health/
Lancet	http://www.thelancet.com
McMaster	http://hiru.mcmaster.c/ebm
Unit for Evidence Based Practice and Policy	http://www.ucl.ac.uk/primcare-popsci/uebpp/uebpp.htm

If you are a BMA member you can have free access to Medline: simply contact the BMA (http://www.bma.org.uk) who will give you your username and password. Some sites act as a 'gateway', which provide a route to further relevant sites.

Two useful 'gateway' sites are:

Wiltshire Health Authority	http://web.ukonline.co.uk/nemisis/index.htm
South West Medical Library	http://www.soton.ac.uk/~swhclu/

By using these 'gateways' you do not have to pay to use the Cochrane database.

The AIRES knowledge finder (http://www.kfinder.com/newweb/) is another useful resource. Although it is very user friendly and enables a user to ask free text questions rather than key words, it is quite expensive.

Other useful websites

National Centre of Clinical Audit	http://ww.uca.org.uk
General Practice On-Line	http://www.priory.com/gp.htm
RCGP	http://www.rcgp.org.uk
WHO	http://www.who.ch/
NEJM	http://www.nejm.org
JAMA	http://www.ama-assn_org/

References

Achterlonie M, Taylor MB (1998) *Taking Control of Learning*. A Small Practices' Association Publication.

Benner, P. (1984) *From Novice to Expert: Excellence and Power in Clinical Nursing Practice*. Addison-Wesley, Harlow.

Bero LA, Grilli R, Grimshaw JM, Harvey E, Oxman A, Thomson MA. (1998) Closing the gap between research and practice: an overview of systematic reviews of interventions to promote the implementation of research findings. *BMJ*; **317**: 465–8.

Carr W (1995) *For Education: Towards Critical Educational Inquiry*. The Open University Press.

Chief Medical Officer (1998) *A Review of Continuing Professional Development in General Practice*. Department of Health, Leeds.

Coles C. (1994) A review of learner-centred education in primary care. *Education for General Practice*; **5**: 19–25.

Institute of Personnel and Development (1997) *Continuing Professional Development*. Institute of Personnel and Development, London.

Curtis AJ. (1998) *Opinion leaders in general practice*. MSc Dissertation, University of Bath.

Department of Health (1998) *A Review of Continuing Professional Development in General Practices. A Report by the Chief Medical Officer*. London: Department of Health.

Eraut M. (1994) *Developing Professional Knowledge and Competence*. Falmer Press, London

Epstein RM. (1999) Mindful practice. *JAMA*; **282**: 833–9.

Fish D. & Coles C. (1998) *Developing Professional Judgement in Health Care: Learning Through the Critical Appreciation of Practice*. Butterworth Heinemann, Oxford.

Freidson E. (1994) *Professionalism Reborn: Theory, Prophecy and Policy*. Policy Press, Bristol.

General Medical Council (1993) *Tomorrow's Doctors: Recommendations on Undergraduate Medical Education*. General Medical Council, London.

Golby M & Parrott A. (1999) *Educational Research and Educational Practice,* Fair Way Publications, Exeter.

Hall M, Dwyer D, Lewis T. (1999) *The GP Training Handbook* (3rd edn) Blackwell Science, Oxford.

Handbook for Practice Management (1999) The Royal Society of Medicine Press, London.

Hiss RG, Macdonald R, Davis WK. (1978). Identification of physician educational influentials in small community hospitals. *Proceedings Seventh Annual Conference in Research in Medical Education*; **17**: 283–8.

Honey P, Mumford A. (1986) *The Manual of Learning Styles*. (Published P Honey, Ardingly House, 10 Linden Ave, Maidenhead, Berks SL6 6HB.)

Kolb, DA. (1985). *Experiential Learning*. Prentice-Hall, London.

Lave J, Wenger E. (1991) *Situated Learning Legitimate Peripheral Participation*. Cambridge University Press, Cambridge.

Lomas, J. (1993). *Teaching Old (and Not So Old) Docs New Tricks: Effective Ways to Implement Research Findings*. McMaster University Centre for Health Economics and Political Analysis. Working Paper 93–94, McMaster University.

Neighbour, R. (1992) *The Inner Apprentice*. Kluwer Academic, London.

NHS (1998) *A First Class Service: Quality in the new NHS*. Department of Health, London.

O'Connell S. (1998) *A Handbook for Non Principals in General Practice*. The Limited Edition Press, Southport.

Piercey ML, Waymouth VW (1998) College of Physicians & Surgeons of British Columbia

Pitts J. (2000) Introducing Clinical Governance–an Educational Basis. *Education for General Practice*. (In press).

Pitts J, Vincent S. (1995) The higher professional education course in wessex–the first year. *Education for General Practice*; **6**: 157–62

Pitts, J. (1994) Audience involvement in a general practice 'refresher course'—the sharing of 'wants' and 'needs'. *Education for General Practice*; **5**: 190–8.

Royal College of General Practitioners (1993) *Portfolio-based Learning in General Practice*. Occasional Paper no. 63. RCGP, London.

Royal College of General Practitioners (1994) *Education and Training for General Practice*. Policy Statement 3. RCGP, London.

Royal College of General Practitioners (1995) *Significant Event Auditing: a Study of the Feasibility and Potential of Case-Based Auditing in Primary Medical Care*. Occasional Paper no. 70. RCGP, London.

Royal College of General Practitioners (1999) *Clinical Governance: Practical Advice for Primary Care in England and Wales*. RCGP, London.

Sackett DL, Richardson WS, Rosenberg W, Haynes RB. (1997) *Evidence Based Medicine: How to Practice and Teach EBM*. Churchill Livingstone, London.

Scally G, Donaldson L. (1998) Clinical governance and the drive for quality improvement in the new NHS in England. *BMJ*; **317**: 61–5.

Secretary of State for Health (1997) *The New NHS: Modern, Dependable*. Department of Health, London.

Schön D. (1984). *The Reflective Practitioner*. Basic Books, New York.

SCOPME (1998a) *Continuing Professional Development for Doctors and Dentists: Recommendations for Hospital Consultant CPD and Draft Principles for all Doctors and Dentists.* Standing Committee on Postgraduate Medical and Dental Education, London.

SCOPME (1998b) *Supporting doctors and dentists at work: an enquiry into mentoring.* Standing Committee on Postgraduate Medical and Dental Education, London.

SCOPME (1999) *Doctors and Dentists: The need for a process of review.* Standing Committee on Postgraduate Medical and Dental Education, London.

Thomsen OO, Wulff HR, Martin A, Singer PA. (1993). What do Gastroenterologists in Europe tell cancer patients? *Lancet*; **341**: 473–6.

Vassilas CA, Donaldson J. (1998) Telling the truth: what do general practitioners say to patients with dementia or terminal cancer? *Br J Gen Pract*; **48**: 1081–2.

While P, Pitts J, Jones P, Ager P, Rowlands S. (1998). Education, Audit and Active Learning: Making the Links? *Education for General Practice*; **9**: 22–9.

Wilkinson E, Bosanquet A, Salisbury C, Hasler J, Boasnquet N. (1999) Barriers and Facilitators to the Implementation of Evidence Based Medicine in General Practice: A Qualitative Study. *Eur J Gen Prac*; **5**: 66–70.

Index

Her Majesty's Stationery Office (HMSO) 167

Institute of Health Service Management 167
Institute of Health Service Managers 167
Internet 158
    useful websites 175
interventions
    effective 68–9
    evaluation 34–5
    planning 30–33
interviews, staff 87–8

JAMA website 175
Joint Committee for Continuing Education of Practice
    Staff 167
Joint Committee for Postgraduate Training for General
    Practice 167
journal clubs 158
journals 68–9, 157–8

keeping up to date 157–8
King's Fund 168
King's Fund Centre 168

Lancet website 175
learning
    CASP workshops 58
    from complaints 74–5
    highlights 125, 128–9
    learning points form 88, 100–101
    lifelong see lifelong learning
    needs see learning needs
    portfolios (educational logs) 4, 9, 10–11
    profiles 44
    self-directed learning groups 156
    styles 10, 44–5
    styles questionnaire 44, 46
learning needs
    identifying 9–11, 84–5, 132–5
    meeting 155–8
    personal 9–11, 125, 136–44
    practice 9–11, 84–5
lifelong learning 4, 9
    non-principals 156
local contacts 174
locums 3, 156
looking after yourself 4, 144–54

McMaster website 175
Macmillan Cancer Relief 168
Manual of Learning Styles 44
Marie Curie Training 168
Medical Defence Union 168
medical ethics 4, 141
Medical Insurance Agency 168
Medical Practices Committee 168
Medical Protection Society Ltd 169
Medical Research Council 169
Medicines Resource Centres (MeRec) 169
Medline 175
Mental Health Act Commission 169
mentoring 155–6
MIND 169
minutes of significant-event audit meetings 66–7
mission statements 114
moral dilemmas 141
multidisciplinary review 44

National Advice Centre for Postgraduate Medical
    Education 169
National Association of GP Tutors 170
National Association of Non-Principals 170
National Association of Patient Participation 170

National Asthma Campaign 170
National Asthma and Respiratory Training Centre 170
National Centre of Clinical Audit website 175
National Counselling Service for Sick Doctors 171
National Deaf/Blind and Rubella Association 172
National Institute for Clinical Excellence 171
National Primary Care Research and Development
    Centre 171
needs
    conflicting 133
    development see learning needs
    educational see learning needs
    health see health needs assessment
    learning see learning needs
    patient's 132–5
NEJM website 175
networks, research 86
NHS Executive 170
no-blame culture 60, 103
non-principals 156

Open University 171

PACT data 3, 81
partner review 103–13
    feedback form 103, 104–7
    plan for continued professional development 103,
        110–13
    procedure 103
    summary record of discussion 103, 108–9
past educational profile 125, 126–7
patients
    communicating audit information 140
    health needs see health needs
    needs 132–5
    simulated 140
Patients Association 173
performance
    indicators 84–5
    management 87, 144, 146–7
Personal Action Plan 88, 98–9
personal development 125–77
Personal Development Plans (PDPs) 3, 9, 159–61
    blind spots 138
    checklist 159
    confidentiality 125
    confidentiality declaration 163
    framework 125–54
    learning highlights 125, 128–9
    learning needs, identifying 9–11, 125, 136–44
    past educational profile 125, 126–7
    PGEA accreditation 125, 138
    proforma 160–61
    SCOT analysis 125, 130–31
    self-audit 125–47
    sticky moments 132–5
personal skills 138
phased evaluation plan (PEP) 138–9
portfolio careers 156–7
portfolios (educational logs) 4, 9, 10–11
Postgraduate Educational Allowance (PGEA) 4
    accreditation 125, 138
practice
    audit 73
    complaints procedure 74–5
    development 58–9
    learning needs 9–11, 84–5
    multidisciplinary review 44
    objectives 120–21
    population, key features 22–3
    population profile 20–21, 78–80
    professional 5, 6–8
    professional development 19–121